Acne

Acne

Diagnosis and Management

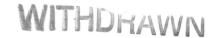

William J Cunliffe MD FRCP
Professor, Department of Dermatology
The General Infirmary at Leeds
Leeds
UK

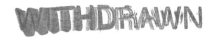

and

Harald PM Gollnick MD
Professor and Chairman, Department of Dermatology and Venereology
Medical Faculty
Otto-von-Guericke-Universität Magdeburg
Magdeburg
Germany

Martin Dunitz

First published in the United Kingdom in 2001 by
Martin Dunitz Ltd
The Livery House
7–9 Pratt Street
London NW1 0AE

Tel: +44-(0)20-7482-2202
Fax: +44-(0)20-7267-0159
e-mail: info.dunitz@tandf.co.uk
Website: http://www.dunitz.co.uk

A CIP catalogue record for this book is available from
the British Library

ISBN 1-85317-206-5

Distributed in the United States by:
Blackwell Science Inc.
Commerce Place, 350 Main Street
Malden MA 02148, USA
Tel: 1-800-215-1000

Distributed in Canada by:
Login Brothers Book Company
324 Salteaux Crescent
Winnipeg, Manitoba R3J 3T2
Canada
Tel: 1-204-224-4068

Distributed in Brazil by:
Ernesto Reichmann Distribuidora de Livros, Ltda
Rua Coronel Marques 335, Tatuape 03440-000
São Paulo
Brazil

Preparation of this book has been supported with a grant from Schering AG, Germany

Composition by Scribe Design, Gillingham, Kent, UK
Printed and bound in Spain by Grafos SA Arte sobre papel

Contents

Preface

The purpose of this book is to provide busy clinicians with an update on the causes of acne. However, much more emphasis is placed on the clinical aspects of acne and its variants. In addition, the therapy of the average patient and the patient whose acne is difficult to treat is discussed in detail. It is also hoped that the illustrations will help to make the book a useful reference in the clinic.

William J Cunliffe
Leeds, UK

Harald PM Gollnick
Magdeburg, Germany

Introduction

Acne is one of the commonest dermatological conditions seen by the practising physician. It typically begins in early adolescence and is frequently associated with other pubertal changes. The age of onset is younger in females, usually around the age of 12 or 13 years of age, and 14 or 15 years in males because of their later onset of puberty. Consequently, the peak incidence of the disease occurs earlier in females, around 17 to 18 years, and in males, around 19 to 21 years.

Acne is frequently associated with a family history, perhaps in up to about 40% of subjects and ongoing research suggests that this may be related also to the type of acne. Different races are affected in different ways. White Caucasians have more acne than black Americans and Japanese have relatively little acne

Acne can be divided into physiological acne, where the patient has a few spots that do not usually need the attention of a physician, and clinical acne occurring in 15% of the population during adolescence, and requiring therapy from a physician.

Treatment for acne may only be required for 3–4 years, but in many patients with obvious clinical acne therapy will be required for 8–12 years until the acne goes into spontaneous remission. Spontaneous remission is usual around the age of 25 years but, in 7%, acne can persist well into the mid-forties or early fifties—the so-called mature acne.

Early recognition and treatment of acne is important to prevent physical scarring and this, along with the inflammatory acne, can be the cause of much psychological distress.

The purpose of this book is to provide the practising physician with a concise overview of acne, the various ways it presents and the optimum treatment of acne patients.

The contents of this book are divided into four sections:

- Pathophysiology of acne;
- Clinical features of acne;
- Acne variants and differential diagnosis;
- Acne therapy, with emphasis on the management of those patients with therapeutically difficult acne.

Although not extensively referenced, some of the more important references will be included for those who are interested in taking the subject further.

Part I: Pathophysiology

1 Sebaceous gland function, physiology and control

Introduction

There is much debate concerning the prime trigger to acne. Is it the increased sebum production or formation of comedones, or could it be that the two abnormalities develop in parallel, possibly in the same acne-prone pilosebaceous follicle?

In this chapter, the factors controlling the sebaceous gland in health and disease are outlined and some clinical entities and therapeutic modulation of the sebaceous gland are discussed.

Histology of the pilosebaceous unit

The pilosebaceous unit comprises an epithelium of mature and developing sebocytes through which the hair and sebum pass (Figure 1.1). Anatomically, the pilosebaceous unit is divided into smaller units, with the upper part the infundibulum and the lower part the acroinfundibulum, the infrainfundibulum, and the sebaceous duct (see Chapter 2).

The sebocytes rest on a basement membrane that is contiguous with the

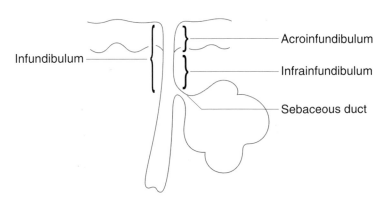

Figure 1.1

Schematic representation of the different anatomical areas of the pilosebaceous unit.

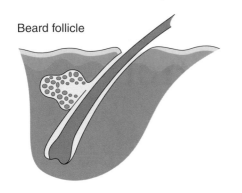

Beard follicle

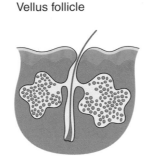

Vellus follicle

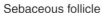

Sebaceous follicle

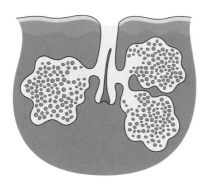

Figure 1.2

The three types of sebaceous gland.

dermis and extend from this basal layer into the central part of the gland. A group of undifferentiated sebaceous gland cells also exist within the more central to lower part of the sebaceous glands; these cells also differentiate to form the typical large fat-laden sebocyte cells. The sebaceous gland is a holocrine gland, i.e. the secretion is the result of self-destruction of the sebocytes. The nucleus is moved to the periphery of the cell. The cells then disrupt, liberating the sebum into a small sebaceous duct, which then enters the pilosebaceous duct. The sebum secreted then moves up with desquamating corneocytes and, where present, microbes to the surface.

Three types of sebaceous gland exist (Figure 1.2).

- Terminal hair-associated gland
- Vellus follicule-associated gland
- Sebaceous follicles.

The terminal hair-associated sebaceous gland follicles are relatively small compared with the sebaceous glands that are involved in acne (the sebaceous follicles) in which the hair is very small compared with its large sebaceous gland. An intermediate form is the vellus follicle-associated gland in which the sebaceous gland is intermediate in size as is the hair follicle that produces several small vellus hairs

Hormonal control of the sebaceous gland

The sebaceous glands produce a considerable amount of sebum in the first 3 months of life, which then gradually reduces to zero at 6 months of age. This neonatal stimulus is likely to be an effect of the fetal and neonatal adrenal androgens. After 6 months of age the sebaceous glands remain quiescent until early adrenarche. At adrenarche, somewhere around 7–8 years, there is an increase in adrenal androgens, in particular dihydroepiandrostenedione, with a resultant increase in sebum excretion. In the early pubertal years there is a further increase in adrenal androgens and gonadal androgen stimulus to the sebaceous gland. There is an obvious increase in greasiness of the skin (seborrhoea), even in subjects who do not have acne. The sebaceous gland is under endocrine control (Figure 1.3). The main stimulus to the sebaceous glands is androgens. The pituitary has an important role in controlling the androgen production via the adrenals and the gonads. The adrenals in particular produce dihydroepiandrostenedione and the gonads in both sexes, testosterone. The circulating androgens, in particular testosterone, are bound to the sex-hormone binding globulin but it is the 1–2% of free testosterone that dictates sebaceous gland activity.

In both sexes, independent of the presence or absence of acne, there is a gradual increase in sebum excretion from puberty and beyond, reaching a peak at about the age of 16–20 years. Thereafter the level remains constant until there is a gradual decrease from about 40 years onwards in women and from about 50 years in males. In general, the sebum excretion rate (SER) in men is significantly higher than in women.

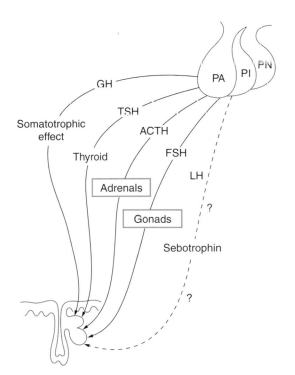

Figure 1.3

Endocrine control of the pilosebaceous gland by the pituitary gland and other intermediate glands.

Sebaceous gland activity and acne

Patients with acne also have seborrhoea; indeed many patients complain that, as acne develops so does an increased greasiness of the skin and of the scalp (Figure 1.4), requiring more regular washing of the face and scalp. There is a reasonable correlation between the amount of sebum produced and the severity of acne. In addition, there is evidence that those subjects with seborrhoea and acne have a higher number of sebaceous lobules per gland. Indeed one of the disappointing features of acne therapy with most therapies is the fact that despite an improvement in the acne the seborrhoea persists. However, with Dianette® and oral

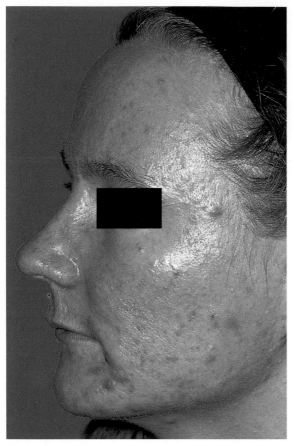

Figure 1.4

Clinical picture of greasy skin in acne.

isotretinoin there is, as the acne improves, a significant reduction in sebum excretion.

Measurements of sebum excretion also show that individuals with acne produce more sebum than individuals who have never had acne (Figure 1.5). Nevertheless, as with control subjects, there is a gradual decrease in sebum excretion beyond the age of about 40 years. Thus reduction in sebum alone does not account for resolution of acne.

Hormonal control of the sebaceous glands in acne

Four possibilities exist to explain the increased production of sebum in acne. There could be an elevated level of circulating hormones caused by: 1. An abnormal pituitary drive; or 2. An abnormal increase in the production of androgens by the adrenals or gonads.

The third possibility is that there is an end-organ hyper-response of the sebaceous glands to normal circulating levels of hormones. Indeed a combination of several factors might be present. What is clinically obvious to all clinicians and acne patients

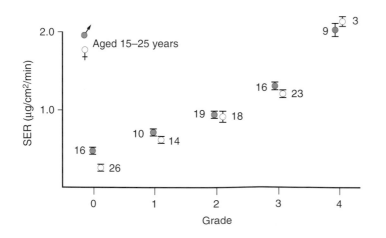

Figure 1.5

Relationship between SER and severity of acne in both males and females.

alike is that acne patients are usually not hormonal misfits. Most females with acne are not excessively hairy, they do not have a hoarse voice, their periods are regular and they get on well with the men and seem to have babies without much difficulty.

There are many investigations, however, showing elevated levels of circulating androgens or an abnormal pituitary drive. Some of these studies, however, have included patients who are older than the typical acne adolescent or who also may have other hormonal problems, such as irregular periods or hormonal misfits. Conversely, in other studies, such changes have been found in the absence of any other obvious clinical androgen. Nevertheless, most patients in the clinic do not require investigations of sex hormones simply because the patients seem otherwise normal, they respond to appropriate treatment reasonably well and thus do not need detailed endocrinological examination. However, there is very little direct evidence confirming an end-organ hyper-response of the pilosebaceous unit to normal levels of circulating androgens. Clinically, physicians will recall seeing many patients with acne just on the face with none on the back and chest or, alternatively, patients with severe acne on the trunk with none on the face (Figure 1.6). This clinical observation

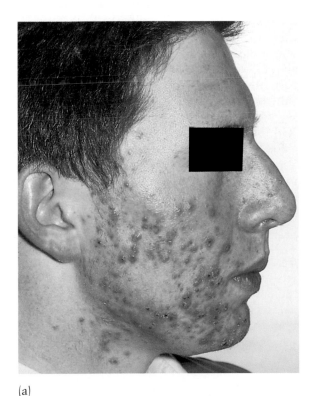

(a)

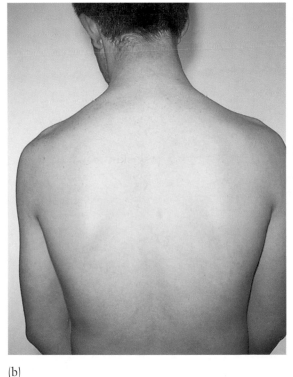

(b)

Figure 1.6

Patient, aged 22 years, with acne for 8 years: (a) face; (b) back. Although the acne is present on the face, none is found on the back. Conversely, acne may be present on the back but not on the face.

supports the likely commonsense logic that the sebaceous glands in acne-prone areas function differently to those in non-prone areas, thus supporting the end-organ hyper-response phenomenon of the sebaceous gland. These clinical observations are supported by experimental data, whereby equipotent amounts of testosterone cream applied to the skin of prepubertal children produced considerable differences in sebum production. Some children produced significantly more sebum than others who had no increase in sebum production (Figure 1.7).

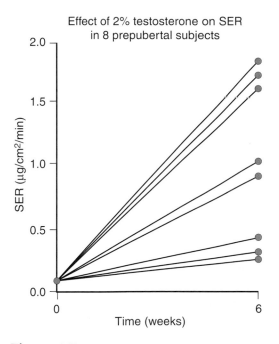

Figure 1.7

Variation in sebum production in prepubertal children after application of testosterone cream to the skin.

Tissue metabolism

Once delivered to the pilosebaceous cells, androgens, especially testosterone are converted to 5-α-dihydrotestosterone (5-α-DHT) by 5-α-reductase type I. Although 5-α-reductase type II is responsible for conversion of testosterone to dihydrotestosterone (DHT) in the hair follicle as well as in the prostate, 5-α-reductase type I has been identified in the sebaceous gland and in the pilosebaceous duct. Figure 1.8 shows a detailed but simplified overview of the intra-cellular metabolism of androgens in the sebaceous gland. It is also likely that 17-β steroid dehydrogenase may also be important in the sebaceous gland; indeed it has been found within the pilosebaceous duct as well as in the sebaceous gland.

Experimentally, immortalized sebocytes can be used to better understand the controlling mechanism of androgens and non-hormonal mechanisms within the sebaceous gland. Studies of in vitro cell culture studies, particularly by Zouboulis and colleagues, have shown that there is considerable intracrine activity controlling androgen metabolism within the skin. In particular the sebaceous gland is pro-androgen active, whereas keratinocytes tend to down-regulate the formation and action of androgens, so producing a controlled androgen environment in and around the pilosebaceous tissues. Variations in this controlling system could explain the different hormonal control of the sebaceous gland cells in patients with acne compared with controls. These in vitro studies support the data derived from observations of individual sebaceous gland activity, which suggests that there is a need to focus on individual sebaceous gland function rather than concentrating too much on the overall rate at which sebum is produced. Different hormonal therapies influence androgenic control of the sebaceous gland in various ways. The effect of different therapies on the pituitary adrenal gonads and the androgen target cell is summarized in Figure 1.9.

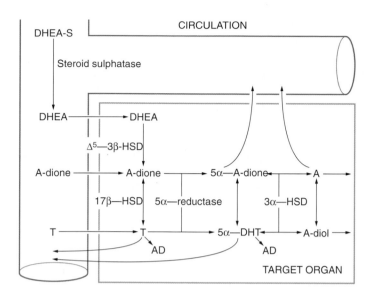

Figure 1.8

Overview of the intracellular metabolism of androgens in the sebaceous gland. AD, androgen receptor; DHEA, dehydroepi-androsterone; DHEA-S, dehydro-epiandrosterone sulphate; Δ^5-3β-HSD, 3β-hydroxysteroid dehydrogenase/ Δ^{5-4}-isomerase; A-dione, androstenedione; 5α-A-dione, 5α-androstenedione; A, androsterone; 17β-HSD, 17β-hydroxysteroid dehydrogenase; 3α-HSD; 3α-hydroxysteroid dehydrogenase; A-diol, androstenediol; 5α-DHT, 5α-dihydrotestosterone; DHT, dihydrotestosterone; T, testosterone. Provided by Professor Zouboulis.

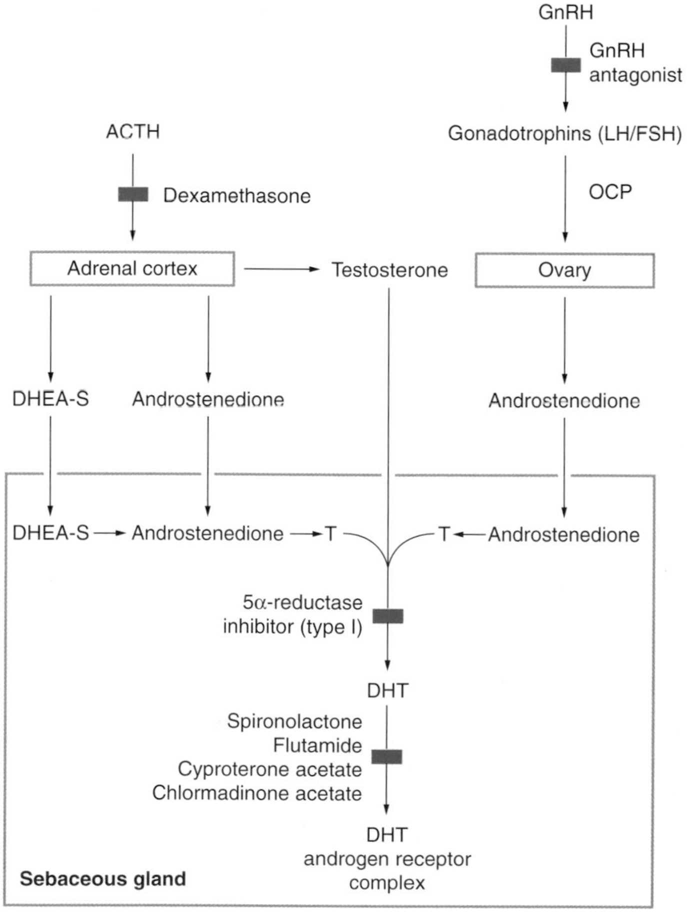

Figure 1.9

Site of action of certain hormone treatments. ACTH, adrenocorticotrophic hormone; DHEA–S, dehydroepiandrosterone sulphate; OCP, oral contraceptive pill; GnRH, gonadotrophin releasing hormones; DHT, dihydrotestosterone.

GnRH

GnRH antagonist

Gonadotrophins (LH/FSH)

ACTH

OCP

Dexamethasone

Adrenal cortex → Testosterone   Ovary

DHEA-S   Androstenedione   Androstenedione

DHEA-S → Androstenedione → T ⟍ ⟋ T ← Androstenedione

5α-reductase inhibitor (type I)

DHT

Spironolactone
Flutamide
Cyproterone acetate
Chlormadinone acetate

DHT
androgen receptor complex

Sebaceous gland

Variability in sebum excretion from different follicles

By applying absorbent paper or tape to a patient's skin, for 30 min, and then staining the skin with a fat stain normal individuals produce an homogenous distribution of sebaceous gland excretion (Figure 1.10a). This is in contrast to subjects with acne who have a wide variation in the pattern of sebaceous excretion from different follicles (Figure 1.10b). Some produce none, some produce a little and some produce a lot. It may well be that certain follicles, possibly those that produce a great deal of sebum, may be the initial trigger to the development of acne lesions. Much work is required on the individual sebaceous gland cell function, allowing us to better understand the relationship between sebaceous gland activity and the development of acne and its subsequent resolution.

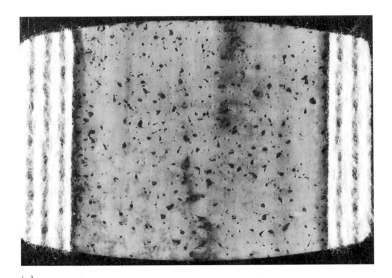

(a)

Figure 1.10

Pattern of sebum excretion determined using Sebotape: (a) in a normal subject; (b) in a patient with severe acne.

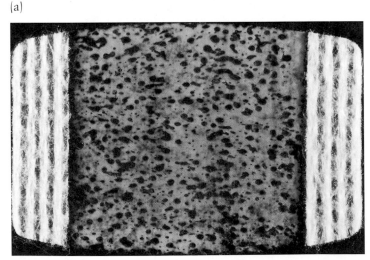

(b)

Methods of measuring sebum excretion rate

Cell culture

Using cell culture, it is possible to separate sebaceous glands and their individual sebocytes and then grow these in vitro. There now exists an immortalized line of sebocytes.

Measurement of overall sebum production using gravimetric technique

Overall sebum production can be measured by using a gravimetric technique in which pre-weighed absorbent papers are placed onto the forehead, the area of which is measured, for 3 hours (Figures 1.11a and b) and then reweighed. Before the clean absorbent papers are applied, it is necessary to pre-clean the

Figure 1.11

Gravimetric technique of measurement of sebum production: (a) papers and gauze are held in position with an elasticated band; (b) final absorbent papers are placed on the forehead using forceps.

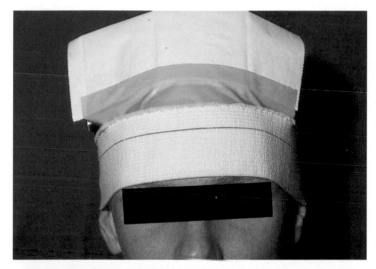

(a)

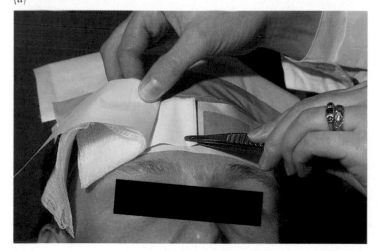

(b)

area by applying similar papers on three occasions each for 15 minutes. This allows the removal of redundant secreted surface lipids. This is perhaps the most precise way of determining sebum excretion but it is time-consuming.

Measuring individual patterns of sebum excretion

These can be measured by using absorbent papers or specially absorbent tapes (Sebotape®) (Figure 1.10), which are applied to the forehead for 30–60 minutes after the skin surface has been wiped with ether or alcohol. It is also possible to semi-quantify the sebum measured using this method, but it is much less reproducible than the gravimetric technique.

Measuring the casual level

It is possible to measure the sebum produced by wiping the forehead with an organic solvent. Variations in the method exist, such as the solvent used and the time the sebum is allowed to accumulate. This technique gives a result that is less reproducible than the gravimetric technique.

Radiolabelling techniques

It is possible to measure the rate of lipid production from the sebocytes by injecting a radiolabelled substrate into the dermis, such as acetate, and measuring the rate of accumulation of radiolabel in the sebum as it emerges from the duct. The sebum can be collected using techniques as described previously. The rate of sebaceous gland cell turnover, that is the rate at which the

sebocyte delivers itself through the holocrine secretion to the surface of the skin, is approximately 21–28 days.

Sebum composition

The composition of sebum is unique to man. This fact might explain, in part, that man is the only species to develop acne. The length and depth of the pilosebaceous unit might also play a role allowing colonization of the duct with *Propionibacterium acnes*, which is an organism not found on any other skin species.

The composition of sebum is also complex. The approximate composition of lipids that is found within the sebocytes and on the surface of the skin is summarized in Table 1.1. The gland itself produces triglycerides, wax esters, squalene and, to a lesser extent, cholesterol and phospholipids. As the sebum moves up the pilosebaceous duct, lipolytic enzymes predominantly from *P. acnes* and *S. epidermidis* convert the triglycerides to free fatty acids. Oxidation of the squalene also occurs as the sebum reaches the skin surface. Thus the surface lipid composition of the skin compared with

Table 1.1   Lipid composition: comparison between isolated sebaceous gland and that on the surface of the skin.

Lipid	% in isolated sebaceous gland	% in skin surface lipids
Triglycerides	56	41
Free fatty acids	0	14
Wax esters	26	26
Squalene	15	16
Cholesterol esters	2	2
Cholesterol	1	1

that of the sebaceous gland shows a reduction in the amount of triglycerides, some mono- and diglycerides and a considerable amount of free fatty acids. Within each group, for example the wax esters, triglycerides and fatty acids, there are also many different chain lengths of fatty acids.

There has been much debate as to the role of sebaceous lipids in health but it is unlikely to be significant, since the skin of youngsters is usually very healthy, requiring no moisturisers or the like. The sebaceous gland is probably an atavistic structure with little or no biological role. Some researchers, however, suggest that colonization of the skin with *P. acnes* which has been found to be immunomodulatory in vivo may endow such a function to the host.

In disease, sebaceous lipids play an important role in the development of acne. Certain lipids are comedogenic; others such as ceramides are decreased. Animal models upon which some of this evidence is based are probably over-predictive; but nevertheless certain fatty acids, squalene and squalene oxide may be important factors in comedogenesis. As described in Chapter 2, a decrease in linoleic concentration may also be important in comedogenesis. Linoleic acid is an essential fatty acid, which enters the sebaceous cells via the circulation and is rate-limited by its concentration in the blood. It is suggested that the linoleic acid is taken up by the sebocytes and that, in large sebaceous glands, there may consequently be a reduction in the sebaceous gland concentration of linoleic acid. This reduced concentration may produce a local deficiency of linoleic acid (LA) in the pilosebaceous duct. Experimentally, animals low in the essential fatty acid, linoleic acid, have a dry skin; resembling the scaliners of a comedone. This is but one possible explanation for comedogenesis. However, despite the persistence of sebaceous gland hyperplasia and deficiency of LA, comedogenesis regresses from the 3rd

decade onwards, as with acne in most of the adolescents.

It has been suggested that certain of the lipids may be important in controlling *P. acnes* growth and certain fatty acids, in particular oleic acid, increase the growth of *P. acnes*. Conversely, certain fatty acids are known to be toxic to bacterial growth and thus the lipid composition may provide some form of bacterial/microbial growth-controlling factors.

Therapeutic modulation of sebum excretion

It is very clear that a significant reduction in sebum excretion rate is associated with clinical improvement (Figure 1.12). Dianette® reduces sebum by 30%. Dianette® plus the anti-androgen cyproterone in a dose-dependent way will further reduce sebum and this is associated with further clinical benefit. Likewise oral isotretinoin in a dose-dependent way will significantly reduce sebum production, and this is associated with a dramatic clinical improvement.

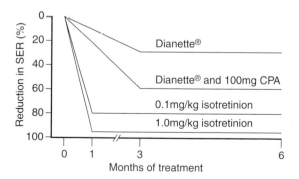

Figure 1.12

The effect of acne therapies in reducing sebum excretion rate (SER).

Changes in sebum rates are also associated with changes in sebum composition, for example both with Dianette® and oral isotretinoin therapy, sebaceous linoleic acid increases as the sebum excretion decreases. This is associated with a reduction in comedone formation. Oral and topical antimicrobials such as benzoyl peroxide, oral and topical antibiotics, significantly reduce free fatty acids by reducing the activity of *P. acnes* lipase and this is associated with clinical improvement.

Resolution of acne

Surprisingly there is very little work on the resolution of acne. Investigations on the resolution of acne need to be performed since such studies could provide useful insight into alternative pharmacological therapies. As acne disappears, there is no reduction in sebum excretion rate until about the age of 40 years. Thus an obvious reduction in sebum excretion is not the explanation for the resolution of acne.

2 Follicular keratinization

Introduction

The pilosebaceous follicles are the target sites for acne (Figure 2.1). It is not known whether the initial trigger for acne is seborrhoea or ductal hypercornification or both. An early initial structural change in acne is the development of comedones, the non-inflamed lesions of acne. Comedones may appear even before teenage years in many acne-prone individuals (Figure 2.2) and they frequently precede inflammatory lesions.

In this chapter, the types of comedones, the histopathogenesis of comedone formation and the factors controlling comedone formation shall be discussed.

Types of comedones

Three major types of comedones exist, namely:

1   Microcomedones
2   Closed comedones (whiteheads)
3   Open comedones (blackheads)

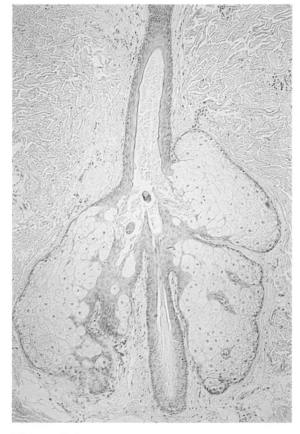

Figure 2.1

Histology of the pilosebaceous gland and pilosebaceous duct typically involved in the acne process.

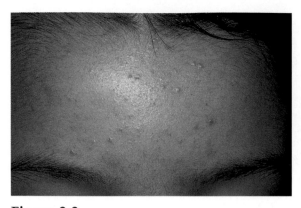

Figure 2.2

Early teenage patient with significant comedones.

Microcomedones

Microcomedones precede any clinical evidence of comedones, the term being purely histological. Early microcomedones are easily recognized as distended pilosebaceous ducts (Figure 2.3). Many microcomedones exist in the apparently normal skin of patients with acne. These microcomedones can be sampled and examined by using a surface biopsy technique. In this technique, cyanoacrylate glue is applied to the skin and a glass slide is pressed on the area for 1 minute (Figure 2.4) and then peeled off.

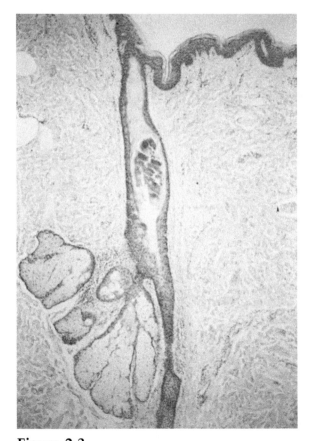

Figure 2.3

Histology of microcomedone formation. Early microcomedones are seen as distended pilosebaceous ducts.

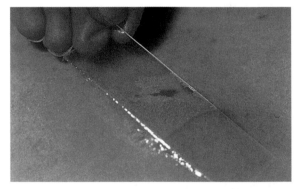

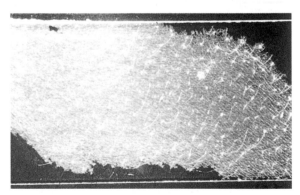

Figure 2.4

Surface biopsy technique of sampling comedones. Cyanoacrolate glue is applied to the skin over which is placed a glass slide. After 1 min the slide is gently peeled off the skin removing with it some of the stratum corneum and comedonal structures.

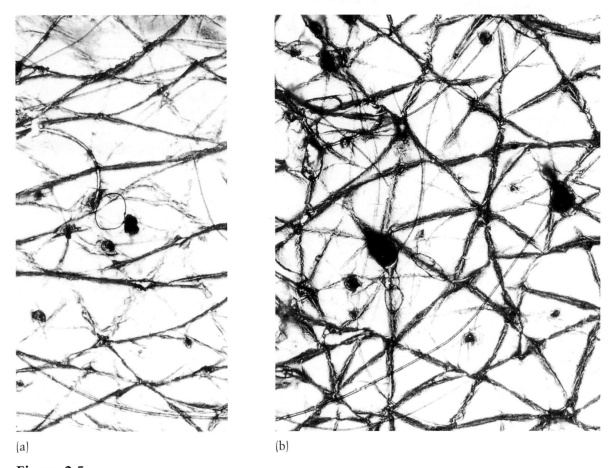

(a)   (b)

Figure 2.5

Dissecting microscopic views of comedones: (a) small follicular cast in mild acne; (b) large follicular casts in severe acne.

Microcomedones remain attached to the slide and can be observed using a dissecting microscope (Figure 2.5). The cyanoacrylate extraction includes the upper part of the pilosebaceous follicles and so it is possible to qualify the microcomedones. This technique has demonstrated that the number of microcomedones increases with disease severity (Figure 2.6).

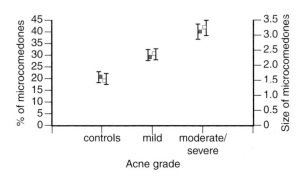

Figure 2.6

Correlation between microcomedones and acne severity.

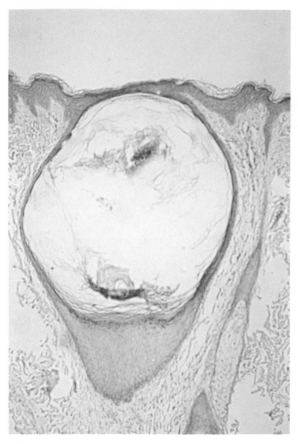

Figure 2.7

Histology of the pilosebaceous duct showing distention with inspissated material typical of a closed comedone (whitehead).

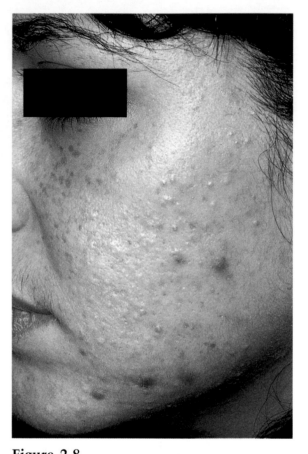

Figure 2.8

Many closed comedones. Note the orifices are barely visible. Also present are some papules.

Closed comedones (whiteheads)

In the closed comedones, the entire pilosebaceous unit is distended with inspissated material (Figure 2.7). The orifice of the closed comedone is barely visible to the naked eye (Figure 2.8). Closed comedones are 0.1–3.0 mm in diameter and are palpable. Some smaller closed comedones may resolve spontaneously within 3–4 days, larger lesions (i.e. macrocomedones or microcysts, Figure 2.9) may be present for many weeks or months. Closed comedones are potentially the most pro-inflammatory of comedones. They are the most frequent non-inflamed clinical lesions, often outnumbering open comedones by a factor of four.

Visualization of closed comedones often requires good light and the use of a ×4 lens. Stretching of the skin (Figure 2.10a and b) enhances the visualization of the closed comedones which may otherwise not be visible. Inability of the physician to identify what can often be many whiteheads may result in inappropriate topical prescribing.

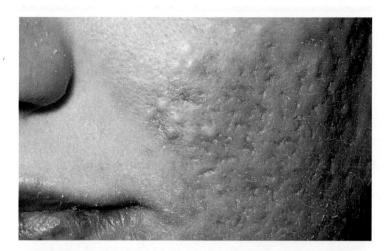

Figure 2.9

Macrocomedone or microcyst: this a closed comedone – larger than 1–5 mm in diameter.

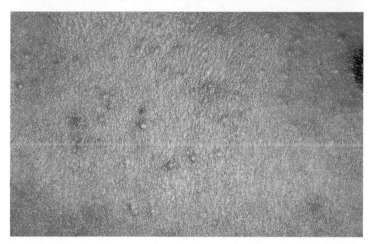

(a)

Figure 2.10

Visualization of closed comedones. (a) Without stretching of the skin only a small number of comedones are seen; (b) stretching the skin demonstrates that there are many comedones present.

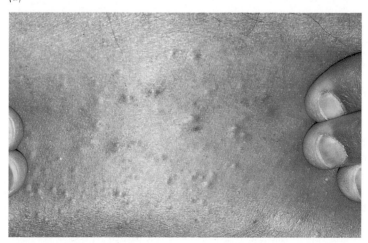

(b)

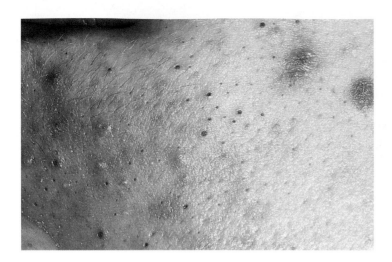

Figure 2.11
Typical blackheads (open comedones).

Open comedones (blackheads)

The open comedone presents clinically as an obvious black lesion, 0.1–3.0 mm in diameter (Figure 2.11). Open comedones usually develop from closed comedones. When a large comedone is expressed with a comedone extractor, the follicular contents are expressed as a pear-shaped, firm grey-white greasy structure. The black tip of the comedone is thought to be caused by melanin rather than oxidation products of comedonal lipids. Although many clinicians regard blackheads as the hallmark of acne, their absence by no means negates the diagnosis. Indeed, there are some acne patients who have few or no blackheads.

- Microcomedones precede clinical comedone formation
- Whiteheads (closed comedones) outnumber blackheads
- 'Normal' looking skin at an acne site is subclinically affected by micro-comedones

---

Histopathogenesis

Acne lesions do not usually occur in a follicle bearing a terminal hair. The hair acts as a wick allowing sebum to drain from the pilosebaceous canal. In contrast, in the pilosebaceous follicles the hairs are small and vellus in nature and often do not reach the surface. They are ineffective wicks and do not therefore prevent the retention of the follicular contents.

Histological examination of the pilosebaceous canal reveals that much of the duct comprises an epidermis-like structure undergoing cornification, the cornified material occupying the more central part of the canal. The upper fifth of the canal, the acroinfundibulum, is very similar to the contiguous epidermis but the lower four-fifths of the canal, the so-called infrainfundibulum (Figure 2.12), is vastly different. In contrast to the overlying epidermis and the epithelium of a terminal hair follicle the infrainfundibulum has an inconspicuous granular layer and an excess of glycogen is often present. The horny cell layers are only a few cells thick and soon desquamate into the central part of the canal to form a heterogeneous mass together with sebum and

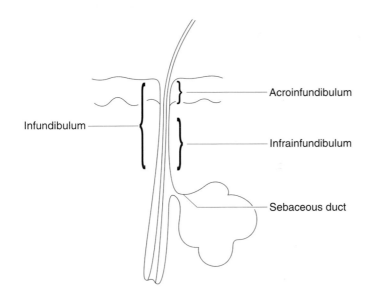

Figure 2.12

Anatomical areas of the pilosebaceous unit. The infundibulum is divided into the acroinfundibulum and infrainfundibulum.

bacteria. The primary site of the developing comedone in the sebaceous follicle in acne vulgaris is at the level of the infrainfundibulum. The granular layer becomes more easily defined; the horny cells become more compact and less readily separable. Similar changes occur also in the small sebaceous ducts, which join the sebaceous gland to the infrainfundibular part of the follicular duct. Thus the horny cells distend the pilosebaceous canal, first producing a microcomedone and then a clinical lesion. It is not known why some lesions remain closed comedones (whiteheads) and why other lesions progress to open comedones (blackheads). As the comedones enlarge, the sebaceous gland may atrophy but sebum continues to be produced until the glands are totally replaced.

Electronmicroscopy shows that in subjects with acne the corneocyte lamellae are thicker, denser and less regular than in those without acne (Figure 2.13).

The follicular cast material (especially the ductal corneocytes) in patients with acne is irregular and arranged in a complex manner. The corneocytes contain lipid droplets not seen in controls (see Figure 2.14). Scanning electronmicroscopy confirms the tortuous

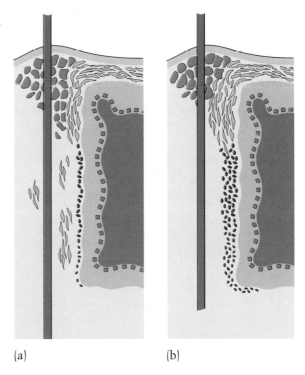

(a)   (b)

Figure 2.13

The corneocyte lamellae. (a) Subject without acne; (b) subject with acne. The corneocyte lamellae are thicker, denser and less regular in those with acne.

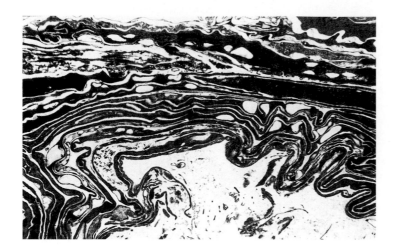

Figure 2.14

Scanning electron microscopy appearance of a pilosebaceous duct showing the interwoven corneocytes.

intertwining of the densely packed corneocytes resembling a rabbit warren (Figure 2.14). This anatomical defect favours retention of sebum and microorganisms between the corneocytes. Compared with a normal follicle, the early comedone has a thickened wall but, as the lesions mature into the microcomedone, the intraluminal contents increase, and there is variable patchy thinning of the ductal wall (Figure 2.15).

> The infrainfundibulum is the site of comedone formation

Evidence for ductal hyperproliferation

The use of labelling, notably thymidine and K_i67 labelling, has produced clear evidence that comedone formation is associated with ductal hyperproliferation. Even without evidence of a microcomedone, some ducts from 'normal' skin in acne-prone areas show evidence of ductal hyperproliferation (Figure 2.15). This is clinically important since it is a reminder that the apparently normal skin of patients should be treated to, hopefully, reduce the rate of formation of new comedones.

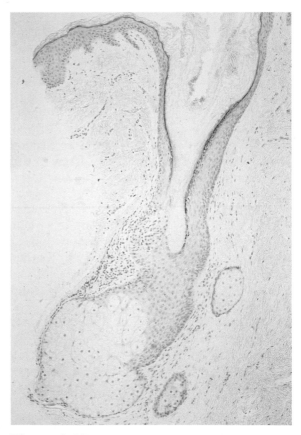

Figure 2.15

Biopsy of an early comedone showing microcomedone formation and variable patchy thinning of the ductal wall.

Evidence for increased cohesiveness of ductal corneocytes

There is no direct evidence for this phenomenon. The histological evidence is suggestive but the mere accumulation of multiple corneocytes in the duct could be caused by either an increase in production of basal corneocytes, which is known to occur, and/or a failure of the corneocytes to be expelled from the duct.

> Comedones represent retention of hyper-proliferating ductal corneocytes

Mechanism of ductal hypercornification

At the molecular level, the reasons for ductal hypercornification are unknown but one or more of several factors might be important:

- Abnormal response to androgen; and/or
- Abnormal lipid composition of the ductal keratinocytes;
- Local cytokine activity; and/or
- Microbial factors

Possible hormonal control of the pilosebaceous duct

Results from in vitro labelling studies may be suggestive of a common controlling mechanism for the sebaceous gland and the pilosebaceous canal. Indeed androgen receptors have been found in both the gland and the pilosebaceous duct. The possibility of a common controlling mechanism is further

supported by the recent work of Thiboutet and colleagues who have shown the presence of 5-α reductase type I in the pilosebaceous duct. Indirect evidence from the use of anti-androgens may also support a role for the androgenetic control of the duct. Patients receiving Diane® and Dianette® show a reduction in comedones (Figure 2.16). This could be a direct anti-androgen effect on ductal corneocytes, or an indirect effect resulting from hormonal-induced changes in sebaceous lipid composition.

> Androgens are likely to be involved in comedogenesis

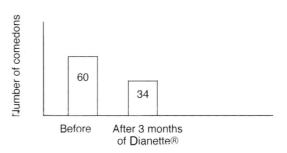

Figure 2.16

Reduction in comedones with Dianette™. A significant reduction is seen.

Lipid changes that might modulate cornification

Role of fatty acids and squalene in inducing comedones

Long-term treatment of acne with clinically effective oral and topical antibiotics is associated with a significant reduction in skin surface lipid free fatty acids. As part of the clinical improvement, there is a reduction in

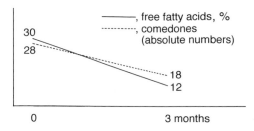

Figure 2.17

Reduction in number of comedones with oral tetracycline (0.5 g bd) therapy. The free fatty acids are also reduced.

the number of comedones (Figure 2.17) and microcomedones. In the mid-1970s it was assumed the follicular free fatty acids triggered off comedogenesis but further human experimental evidence lay some doubt on this issue.

Squalene, in particular its oxide, has also been implicated as a possible cause of comedogenecity. The surface lipids of patients with acne have an increased squalene content compared with controls. In the rabbit ear, squalene is comedogenic. The degree of hypercornification produced in the rabbit ear by components of sebum is related to concentration. The percentage of each component of sebum needed to elicit a response in the rabbit ear in most instances exceeds normal levels in human sebum.

The comedogenicity of UVA-irradiated and non irradiated substances (squalene, oleic acid, isopropyl nyristate, squalene and liquid paraffin) has also been investigated in rabbits using surface microscopy and histological examination. Squalene peroxides were highly comedogenic. Both oleic acid and its peroxides were able to induce fairly large comedones and there was good correlation between the lipid peroxide levels and the size of the comedones. Animal models of comedone formation may be overpredictive

and may, however, not strictly relate to comedone formation in man.

Role of linoleic acid in inducing comedones

A link between comedogenesis and a low sebum level of linoleic acid was proposed by Downing and co-authors. They found that patients with acne had a significantly lower level of linoleic acid in their skin surface lipids than normal individuals. Subsequent studies have suggested that this effect relates to the higher sebum secretion rates characteristic of acne, since there is an inverse relationship between the secretion rate and the linoleate content of the surface wax esters, which are purely of sebaceous origin. Conversely, a reduction in the rate of sebum secretion by treatment with the anti-androgen cyproterone acetate, or with oral isotretinoin, causes a corresponding increase in the linoleic acid content of the sebaceous lipids.

Linoleic acid is an essential fatty acid. It is proposed that, at the time of cell division, when the sebaceous cells still have contact with the basement membrane, they still have access to circulating lipids, including linoleate. Once sebum synthesis begins, no further lipids are accepted from the circulation, so that the more sebum that is synthesized per cell, the more the initial linoleate content will be diluted. This linoleate will be released at the time of final cell rupture and incorporated into various lipids in proportion to the relative rates at which these lipids are being synthesized at the time of cell rupture.

It is proposed that when the secretion rate of sebum is high, as in acne, and, as a result, its linoleate concentration is low, the cells of the follicular epithelium might thereby be subjected to lipids that are deficient in essential fatty acids. Support for this hypothesis has been further obtained by examination of the polar lipids recovered from comedones, the acyl ceramides of which contained only 6% linoleate among the esterified fatty acids, compared with 45% in the acyl ceramides from normal human epidermis. These data can be taken as an indication of essential fatty acid deficiency in the comedo-forming epithelial cells in which the acyl ceramides were synthesized.

The characteristic findings in animals with essential fatty acid deficiency are epidermal hypercornification and decreased epidermal barrier function. Similarly, a low lineolate concentration in the follicles of patients with acne could contribute to the corneocyte impaction that constitutes comedone formation, as well as to make the follicular wall more permeable to pro-inflammatory factors. However, there is some debate concerning this hypothesis. For example, despite ongoing seborrhoea in the third and fourth life decade, acne is decreasing in parallel.

An alternative suggestion for ductal cornification is the possibility that the high sebum flow in acne-prone follicles produces a local deficiency of vitamin A in the duct.

- It is likely that lipid composition influences comedone formation
- A low sebum linoleate is in particular likely to be important
- Other lipids, such as squalene, or fatty acids, or their peroxides and low ceramides may play a role

---

Cytokine control of comedone formation

Investigations by Keeley and colleagues have shown that cytokines significantly influence comedone formation. In vitro studies demonstrated that IL-1α added to cultured ducts induced the development of comedones (Figure 2.18a). This process could be blocked by IL-1 antagonists. Furthermore, formation was totally disrupted by epidermal growth factor (EGF) (Figure 2.18b)

Cytokines do influence comedone formation

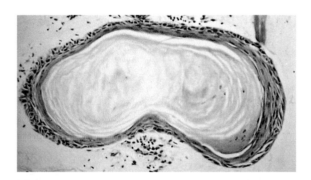

(a)

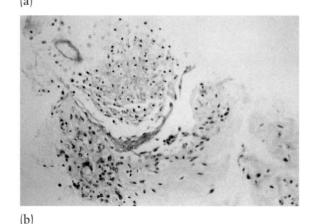

(b)

Figure 2.18

Development of comedones induced in vitro (a) by IL-1α added to cultured ducts in vitro. (b) Similar follicles to (a) to which have been added EGF. Courtesy of T Keeley, Cambridge.

The relationship between bacteria and abnormal ductal cornification

Two studies have failed to incriminate bacteria in the initiation of comedones. Firstly, ultrastructural studies have shown that some early comedones do not contain bacteria. Secondly, cultures of some early non-inflamed biopsy material taken from lesions are sterile (Figure 2.19).

However, effective antimicrobial therapy may decrease comedones, even at 4 weeks of therapy. Comedo reduction occurs with oral and topical antibiotics, and other antimicrobial agents such as benzoyl peroxide.

Although this could be a direct effect resulting from a modulation of comedogenesis, a more tenable explanation is that it results from an indirect effect on sebum composition. Thus, it is probable that the early hypercornification of acne is not initiated by bacteria, but antimicrobial factors may later inhibit bacterial lipases, so reducing sebaceous free fatty acids.

> • *P. acnes* is not involved in the initiation of comedones but may be involved in later stages of comedogenesis
> • Antimicrobial therapies for acne may reduce existing comedones

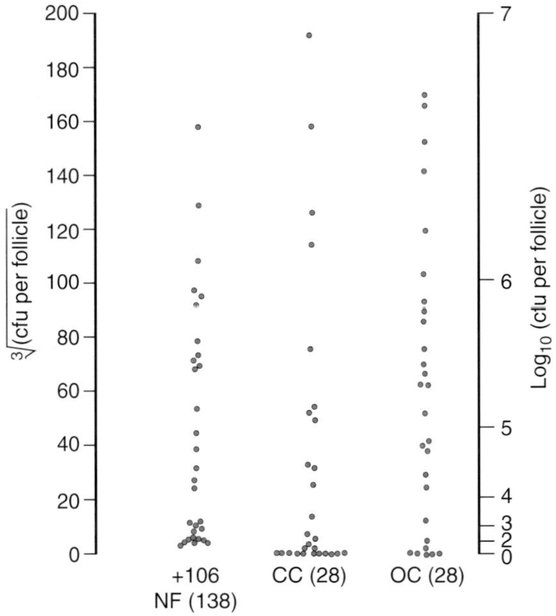

Figure 2.19

Bacterial densities in cultured biopsy material from early non-inflamed comedones: a comparison with normal pilosebaceous follicles. This shows that some biopsies of early comedones are sterile, that is, no bacteria are present. NF, Normal follicles; CC, Closed comedones; OC, Open comedones.

Trigger factors for acute ductal obstruction

Corneocytes usually contain about 20% water but this varies markedly with age. The swelling of the epidermis caused by hydration that follows prolonged soaking of the skin, particularly in warm water, is familiar to most people. There is nothing to suggest that the pilosebaceous duct corneocytes are spared such an effect. It seems reasonable, therefore, to suggest that if the cornified epithelium of the sebaceous follicle becomes hydrated, this might increase sebum outflow resistance by reducing the size of the pilosebaceous ostium. Acute obstruction of a particular pilosebaceous duct may then occur and thus precipitate acne. The hydration effect has been proven in subjects with acne (Figure 2.20). This has clinical implications, for example acne is a feature in patients working in hot humid environments, following adhesive plaster occlusion and when an individual goes from a temperate to a humid

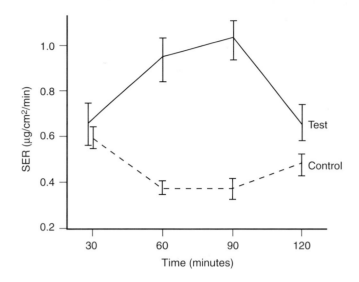

Figure 2.20

Sebum excretion rate at 30 min intervals after removal of occlusion which had been in place for 22 h. Note on the test (occluded) site that there is an increase in sebum outflow compared with the control (non-occluded) site suggesting that on the test side the occlusion (hydration) clamps back the sebum which subsequently 'escapes' on relieving the hydration.

environment such as the Mediterranean areas in summer.

> • Relative acute changes in skin hydration and oily sunscreens may precipitate acne, producing 'acne Mallorca'

Resolution of comedones

It is not widely recognized that comedones may undergo spontaneous resolution. Clearly this must happen, otherwise an individual with acne would, after only a few years, have many comedones. Time studies observing such a phenomenon have shown that many whiteheads resolve spontaneously without treatment after about 8 days. A better understanding of this phenomenon might help better treatment of comedones. It is also perhaps pertinent to note that mature individuals who now no longer have acne may have a seborrhoea but they usually do not have comedones.

> • Investigations on the natural resolution of comedones may help in a better treatment for reducing comedones

3 Microbiology of acne

Introduction

The limited species of organisms that colonize the skin surface include bacteria such as propionibacteria, staphylococci and aerobic coryneform bacteria and the yeast *Malassezia furfur* (Figures 3.1–3.3). In addition to these resident organisms other microorganisms appear and disappear from the skin environment and constitute transient flora. Staphylococci are the first organisms to colonize the skin, but an individual's resident microflora develops over time and the full range of the resident microflora does not develop definitively until puberty. At that time, in skin sites with a high number of sebaceous follicles, the measurable microbial population may reach levels of 10^7 organisms/cm^2. Thereafter the microflora density remains constant until it starts to decrease in old age.

All resident microflora possess attributes that enable them to colonize human skin. They possess a thick, structurally strong cell

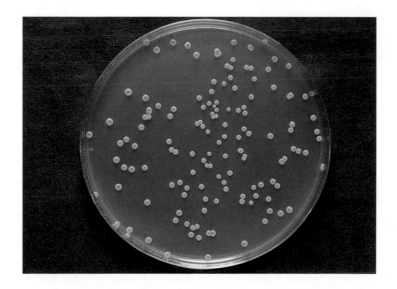

Figure 3.1

Colony appearance of the propionibacteria, *P. acnes*. (Courtesy of Professor KT Holland.)

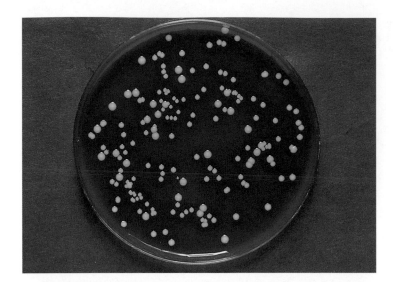

Figure 3.2

Colonies of *Staph. epidermis* (grey/white) and *M. luteus* (yellow) on heated blood agar. (Courtesy of Professor KT Holland.)

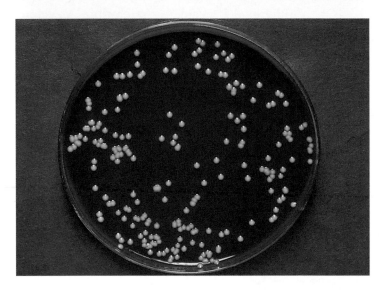

Figure 3.3

Colonial appearance of *M. furfur*. (Courtesy of Professor KT Holland.)

wall, which assists in protecting the microflora against drying from external osmotic pressure. They are non-motile and possess extracellular enzymes that can degrade some of the relatively insoluble skin polymers on the skin surface, for example lipids. *Propionibacterium acnes*, the predominant follicular resident organism, is likely to be involved in the aetiology of acne, partic-ularly inflammatory acne, and possibly involved in the later stages of comedo forma-tion. Acne is not, however, an infectious disease, and only very occasionally are the transient flora involved in acne. The best example of transient organism involvement of an acne-related disease is in Gram-negative folliculitis (Figure 3.4). This is a rare true bacterial folliculitis resulting from the

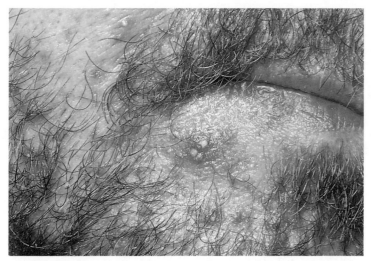

(a)

Figure 3.4

Gram-negative folliculitis. (a) The face of a patient who had been taking tetracycline therapy for 9 months. (b) Close-up view of Gram-negative folliculitis showing the presence of many pustules.

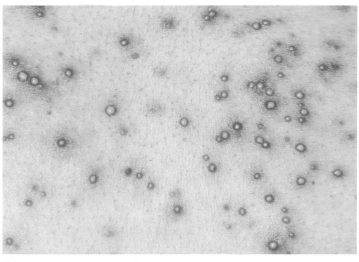

(b)

seeding of organisms from the anterior nares onto the adjacent skin after the resident flora is suppressed by long-term systemic or topical antibiotics.

The aim of this chapter is to review the evidence incriminating *P. acnes* in the aetiology of acne. The effect of therapy on *P. acnes* on the skin, and *P. acnes* resistance will be discussed, as will microbiology of Gram-negative folliculitis.

> • Acne is not infectious but its development is likely to be linked with the commensal *P. acnes*

General description of *P. acnes*

In the pathogenesis of acne, the most important organism is *P.acnes*. These organisms are Gram-positive, non-motile rods that tend to be irregular when first isolated and are sometimes short-branching. During laboratory culture, a relatively easy process, the bacterial cells become more regular and smaller. Isolation requires 7 days of incubation under anaerobic conditions at 35–37°C (however, the organisms are not strict anaerobes). Depending on the species, the colonies are buff-pink, and are generally dome-shaped. Although several species of propionibacterium exist, *P. acnes* is the important organism in acne.

P. acnes is non-motile and the mode of penetration of the follicular duct is unknown but may relate to the physiological microenvironment of the follicule and its microenvironmental adaptation.

The physiological microenvironment of the follicle and the microenvironmental adaptation of *P. acnes* may be important factors in the penetration of this non-motile bacterium into the follicular duct

---

Physiology of *P. acnes*

Little information is known about the precise microenvironment of *P. acnes* other than the knowledge that the area is very lipid rich. The organisms are non-motile, so it is unknown how they reach the depths of the follicle. Like most bacteria, *P. acnes* requires a nitrogen source, this being derived not from sebum but from corneocytes. Conversely carbon and hydrogen may be obtained from both lipids and corneocytes. *P. acnes* uses carbohydrates as the carbon energy source, but also requires amino acids and specific vitamins, for example biotin, nicotinic acid and thiamine. The growth and enzyme function of *P. acnes* is greatly influenced by pH and oxygen tension (Figures 3.5 and 3.6). In vitro requirements

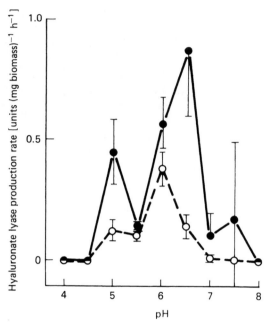

Figure 3.5

Graph showing the effect of pH on two enzymes produced by *P. acnes*. (Courtesy of Professor KT Holland.)

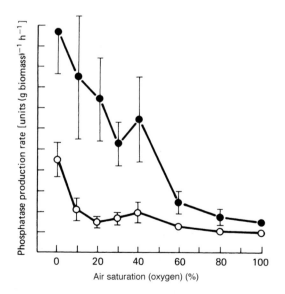

Figure 3.6

Graph showing the effect of oxygen tension on the one enzyme produced by *P. acnes*. (Courtesy of Professor KT Holland.)

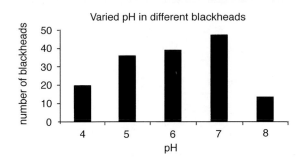

Figure 3.7

The variation in pH of blackheads.

have shown great variation in the growth rate and enzyme production by *P. acnes* under differing oxygen tensions and pH values; moreover the pH of blackheads, at least, varies enormously (Figure 3.7), thus influencing the growth and enzyme production of its resident bacteria. The organisms have optimum growth in the temperature range 30–37°C, temperatures that are likely to be found in the follicle.

Exoenzyme production

P. acnes produces many exoenzymes. The precise function of the exoenzymes in vivo is unknown, although lipases may play a role in the pathogenesis of acne. Production of these enzymes is sensitive to local pH and oxygen tension, although the enzymes so far studied appear to have stabilities and activities that are suited to the optimum pH range for organism growth under slightly acidic conditions (pH 5–6.5), as found on the skin surface. In contrast to the skin surface, however, there may be variations in the follicular environment owing to variations in duct size and sebum flow. The microenvironmental variations in individual follicles could explain the enhanced proliferation or

biological activity of *P. acnes* in one follicle in favour to an adjacent follicle.

> • The growth and function of *P. acnes* relate to its physiological requirements which must mirror its environment

Distribution, density and location of the cutaneous flora

There are many ways of sampling cutaneous bacterial flora.

Surface swab sampling

Taking surface swabs is the easiest method, providing bacterial samples adequate for determining resistance patterns. Using this technique, however, precise information on numbers of organisms cannot be obtained.

Surface scrub techniques

Surface scrub techniques provide information on the level of colonization on the surface of the skin. A standard volume of sampling fluid, such as Triton, is placed within the confines of a metal ring and the skin is gently rubbed with a Teflon rod for 2 minutes. The sampling fluid is then processed using accepted biological techniques.

Using surface scrubs, it can be shown that *P. acnes* is distributed in greater numbers at skin sites where high numbers of sebaceous follicles are found. Staphylococci are found at the same sites but in lower densities. It can also be shown that, accompanying the onset of acne at puberty, there is a large increase in the population of *P. acnes* and only a small increase in the *Staphylococcus* spp. population. Another useful procedure is to use the surface biopsy technique. With surface biopsies it is possible to sample organisms from the upper parts of the duct. There is no relationship between the surface numbers of *P. acnes* and the severity of acne. This is probably because samples are obtained from many follicles, masking a high organism density from one follicle and a low-level colonization of other follicles.

Biopsy and culture of specific follicles

The most informative technique (but the most difficult) is biopsy and culture of specific follicles. It would be most pertinent to obtain biopsies from affected sebaceous follicles or, preferably, the sebaceous follicle that is about to be involved in an acne event, which is impossible to predict.

Using the biopsy procedure, it has been shown that 'normal' follicles are infrequently colonized; 80% of early comedones are colonized and almost all early inflammatory lesions are colonized (Figure 3.8). Colonization is by the two bacterial species, *P. acnes* and *S. epidermis*, and by the yeast *M. furfur*.

There is also variation in the distribution of organisms within the follicle. The *P. acnes* organisms have a restricted distribution compared with the staphylococci. *P. acnes* is found deep in the follicle and more centrally, an environment less variable and more suitable for the more demanding *P. acnes*. *M. furfur* is usually found close to the surface.

- Surface swabs are useful for assessing *P. acnes* resistance
- Follicular sampling, especially single follicle sampling, is the best method for investigating the role of *P. acnes* in acnegenesis

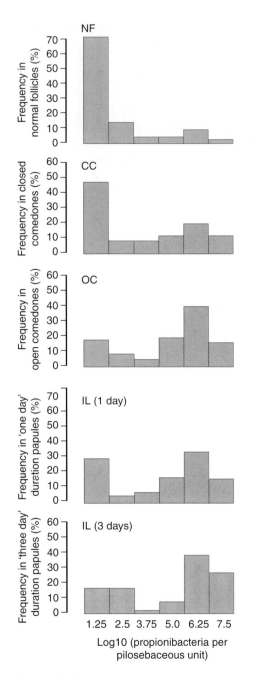

Figure 3.8

Distribution of propionibacteria in normal follicles (NF), open comedones (OC), closed comedones (CC) and early (1 day) and older (3 days) inflamed lesions (I) from the back. (Courtesy of Professor KT Holland.)

The importance of *P. acnes* in acne

Two major facts support the role of *P. acnes* in acne. Firstly, there is a correlation between the reduction in number of *P. acnes* and clinical improvement in patients adequately treated with antimicrobial agents. Secondly, there is some correlation between the flares of acne and the presence of antibiotic-resistant *P. acnes* organisms.

P. acnes has been thought by many to be a major causative actor in inflammatory acne. In view of this, a relentless search has been mounted, and no doubt will continue, to find the acnegenic determinants of this organism. These studies have demonstrated that there is a range of biologically active exoproducts of *P. acnes* such as lipases, proteases, hyaluronidase and characteristic factors that are pro-inflammatory. There is much less evidence to link the microflora to the production of comedones.

- There is a correlation between the reduction in *P. acnes* counts and the clinical improvement in acne
- The development of resistance to *P. acnes* may equate with clinical failure to treat the acne

---

Nasal carriage of *P. acnes*

It is now recognized that *P. acnes* frequently, and in high numbers, colonize the anterior nares. Whether colonization at this site precedes the development of acne or whether it occurs after the onset of the disease is unknown.

- The significance of nasal colonization of *P. acnes* is unknown

---

Folliculitis

It is not the purpose of this chapter to present a discussion of bacterial folliculitis, which is caused by *S. epidermidis*. Nevertheless, two types of folliculitis, Gram-negative folliculitis and Pityrosporum folliculitis, should be discussed here.

Gram-negative folliculitis

Gram-negative folliculitis is an infrequent, but potentially difficult-to-treat, complication of long-term antibiotic treatment, particularly long-term oral therapy. Antibiotics significantly change the normal follicular microbial population and in this situation, Gram-negative bacteria, which probably are seeded from the nares, colonize the follicles. It has been suggested that not only does the antibiotic treatment reduce the normal skin flora, but treatment changes the nasal flora allowing Gram-negative bacteria to colonize this site, too. It is also possible that genetically determined host factors may be important in the bacterial colonization of the follicles. Approximately 80% of patients with cases of Gram negative folliculitis present with superficial pustules, while the remaining patients present with deep nodules and pustules. The possibility of a Gram-negative folliculitis should be entertained if a patient develops a highly inflamed flare after doing well on antibiotics. If clinically suspected, persistent lesions should be sampled and cultured. Organisms isolated include *Escherichia*, *Klebsiella*, *Serratia*, *Pseudomonas* and *Proteus* species. Swab samples from the nose should also be examined for these bacteria. Proteus species are more prevalent in superficial folliculitis rather than with deeper lesions. Once established, these bacteria are difficult to eliminate and antibiotic therapy with ampicillin 0.5 g bd or trimethoprim 400–600 mg/day directed towards these organisms is sometimes successful. The preferred therapy is, however, the use of oral isotretinoin (0.5–1.0 g/day) for 4 months. Such therapy works by altering the microenvironment of the pilosebaceous duct. Relapse may occur but retreatment with oral isotretinoin is usually predictable and successful.

Pityrosporum folliculitis

Pityrosporum folliculitis has been documented as a separate disease (Figure 3.9), with its diagnosis based on clinical appearance and the abundance of pityrosporum yeasts (*M. furfur*) in the follicles. It has been shown, however, that the incidence and density of *M. furfur* on normal back skin is a feature of 75% of normal follicles. Therefore, at present, the view that *M. furfur* alone causes folliculitis must be questioned. Several explanations could account for apparently conflicting data. Folliculitis may occur for three reasons:

1   The follicular population of *M. furfur* exceeds a high but crucial number or the folliculitis is caused by specific biovar of *M. furfur*.
2   The folliculitis may occur when the follicular environment changes to a unique set of conditions that encourages the microorganisms to produce the pathogenic determinants involved in the disease.
3   The folliculitis may occur because of any combination of 1 or 2.

Future investigations, especially directed towards analysis of *M. furfur* variation of isolates, should help to resolve the role and importance of this micro-organism in pityrosporum folliculitis.

- The microbiology of normal follicles, acne-affected follicles and pityrosporum folliculitis is similar. It is limited to a narrow range of micro-organisms (propionibacteria, staphylococci and *M. furfur*)
- Circumstantial evidence incriminates *P. acnes* in inflammatory acne. The extent of involvement of *P. acnes* is still under investigation, as is the specific mechanism by which it exerts its effects
- With regard to Gram-negative folliculitis, there is irrefutable evidence proving that the Gram-negative bacteria are not found in normal follicles, but are present only in these pathologically affected follicles

---

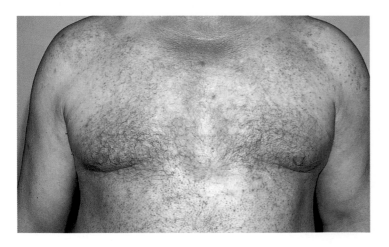

Figure 3.9

Patient with ill-defined erythematous occasionally pustular papules of pityrosporum folliculitis.

4 Acne inflammation

Morphogenesis of inflammatory acne lesions

To the patient, the inflammatory lesions of acne are usually the most important. There are several possible presentations.

The inflamed lesions are polymorphic and may be divided into lesions that are superficial:

- Papules (Figure 4.1)
- Pustules (Figure 4.2) and
- Macules (Figure 4.3)

and those lesions which develop deep or within the skin:

- Nodules (Figure 4.4)
- Deep pustules (Figure 4.4)

It is generally accepted that the majority of inflamed lesions develop from microcomedones, although both open and closed comedones and normal follicles may also become inflamed. Investigations on the clinical development of inflamed lesions are difficult to perform because they involve several visits by patients to the clinic for observation. The data available indicates that inflamed lesions develop dynamically, with

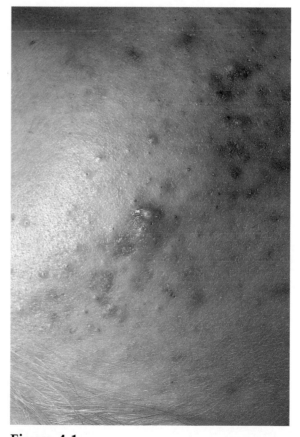

Figure 4.1

Papules and pustules, some of which are arising from whiteheads.

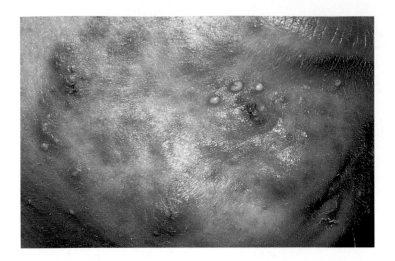

Figure 4.2

Typical pustules and deep nodular lesions.

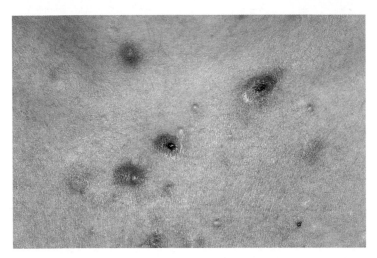

Figure 4.3

Papular lesions resolving into macules.

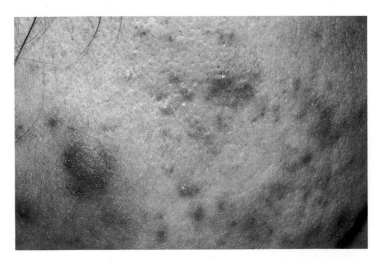

Figure 4.4

A patient with a nodule (left) and some small papules. Also present are some hyperpigmented macules (right).

the majority exhibiting polymorphic, clinical and histological appearances before resolving. For example a papule may become pustular before resolving, usually through a macular phase. Over 50% of superficial lesions resolve within 7–10 days, whereas the deep-seated nodules and pustules may persist for 10–30 days or even longer.

- Superficial acne lesions persist for up to 10 days
- Deeper lesions persist for up to 30 days or longer

Histology of inflamed lesions

The time relationships in acne inflammation are summarized in Table 4.1.

Early events

Historically there was controversy regarding the initial events that occur in the development of inflammation in acne. One school of thought favoured the view that inflammation commenced with focal infiltrates of mononuclear cells (e.g. lymphocytes and monocytes/macrophages), whereas Kligman proposed that neutrophil polymorphonuclear leucocytes were the predominant cell type in early foci of inflammation. Kligman's observations profoundly affected research in the field of acne inflammation throughout the 1970s and early 1980s, which attempted to take account of the neutrophil in the initiation of the inflammatory response. The resultant popular opinion held that chemotactic factors produced by bacteria in the pilosebaceous duct lumen were able to diffuse out of the follicle into the dermis and attract neutrophils to the site. The neutrophils then brought about disruption of the follicle wall. This in turn facilitated the leakage of comedonal material (e.g. bacteria, ductal corneocytes and sebum) into the dermis.

The controversy regarding the initial events in the inflammatory process arose because of the difficulties in interpreting dynamic processes by histological examination of static biopsy material. In 1988, Norris and Cunliffe published the results of a study that addressed two important questions: the

Table 4.1   The likely development of inflammation in papular acne lesions.

Stage	Cell	Likely stimulus
Non-inflamed	—	IL-α
Very early (6 hours)	CD4$^+$ T-lymphocytes	Endothelial cell I-cam E-selectin
Early (24–48 hours)	CD4$^+$ T-lymphocytes Neutrophils	I-cam E-selectin *P. acnes* Chemotaxins
Middle/late (72 hours plus)	CD4$^+$ T-lymphocytes Macrophages Giant cells	*P. acnes* and other microbes 'Free' corneocytes, keratins

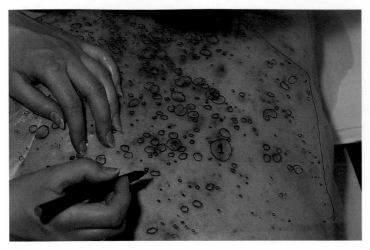

(a)

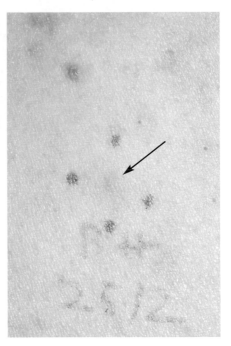

(b)

Figure 4.5

(a) An acne patient whose spots and reference points have been marked onto a cellulose acetate sheet. (b) Using this technique an early inflamed lesion can be detected 6 hours after the original template was used.

identity of the initial inflammatory cell; and whether duct rupture was necessary for the development of inflammation. The authors used a lesion mapping technique, which enabled them to take biopsies of 'timed' lesions undergoing inflammatory changes (Figures 4.5a and b). In all, 69 early inflamed papular lesions were studied. In most studied at 6 and 24h there was a focal perivascular and periductal mononuclear cell infiltrate (Figures 4.6 and 4.7). Neutrophils were only observed in later lesions (over 48 h) and were most evident when there was a concomitant disruption of the pilosebaceous follicle wall (Figure 4.8). Importantly, disruption of the duct wall was only observed in 14% of 6 hour old inflamed lesions and 23% of 72 hour old inflamed lesions (Figure 4.9). The authors concluded that the initial infiltrate in inflamed lesions was mononuclear and that the cells infiltrated in the absence of gross structural damage to the pilosebaceous follicle wall (Figure 4.8). Neutrophils were observed in the pustular lesions.

- Lymphocytes are the first cell type in papules
- Duct disruption is not a prime event in the development of papules

---

The initial events in inflammation in acne have been studied further and in detail using immunocytochemistry to identify the phenotype of the cells involved and the expression of markers of cell activation in 'timed' lesional biopsies. The predominant cells in initial perivascular and periductal focal infiltrates have been shown to be CD4$^+$ T-lymphocytes (T-helper cells). The endothelial cells lining periductal blood vessels have been demonstrated to express high levels of the vascular adhesion molecules, V-cam and

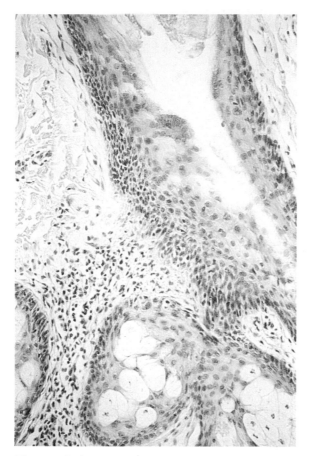

Figure 4.6

A very early papule. Note the appearance of a little oedema and mononuclear cell infiltrate.

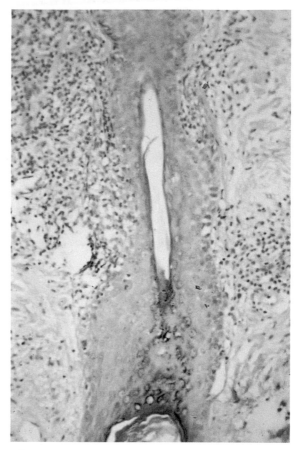

Figure 4.7

A later stage papule (12–24 h). Note the appearance of more mononuclear cells and more oedema.

E-selectin. In addition, the cellular infiltrate, endothelial cells and cells in the duct wall have been shown to express high levels of HLA-DR (MHC Class II – a marker that the cells are activated) in 6-hour-old inflamed lesions. These findings indicate that the inflammatory changes in acne are initiated by the up-regulation of vascular adhesion molecules on dermal endothelial cells periductally leading to an accumulation of mononuclear cells, which are predominantly CD4+ T-lymphocytes.

> • T-helper cells are the most predominant lymphocyte in acne (papular) inflammation

Current research into the mechanisms of inflammation in other dermatoses, for example psoriasis and contact dermatitis, has indicated important unifying concepts. It has been proposed that T cells will migrate independently of antigen into the dermis

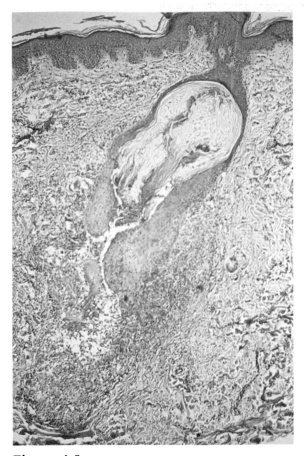

Figure 4.8

A pustular lesion demonstrating disruption of the pilosebaceous duct and many polymorphs.

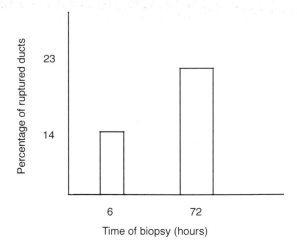

Figure 4.9

The relationship between the time of an inflamed lesion and ductal rupture. It is clear that ductal rupture is not an early event in acne inflammation.

following release of pro-inflammatory cytokines by keratinocytes which up-regulate vascular adhesion molecule expression. The initiation of antigen-independent cutaneous inflammation may then promote an antigen-dependent amplification phase via antigen-dependent T-cell responses. The histological features of both early inflammatory acne lesions and established inflammatory acne lesions are in keeping with these concepts.

Late events

Histologically, late inflammatory lesions demonstrate a chronic cellular infiltrate consisting of lymphocytes, macrophages (histiocytes) and some giant cells (Figure 4.10). Neutrophils, when present, are invariably located within and around the pilosebaceous duct lumen, the site where bacteria are located. The severity of the lesion is dependent upon the degree of structural damage to the pilosebaceous duct wall and the length and level of exposure of the dermis to follicular contents. Histologically deep seated nodular lesions resemble foreign-body type granulomatous reactions with the offending agents thought to be corneocytes and bacteria.

Inflammatory lesions resolve via a macular phase. Histologically, macules show a predominantly lymphocytic and histiocytic infiltrate that slowly resolves over 2–48 days depending on the initial severity of the

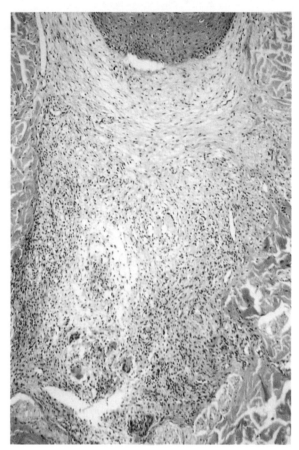

Figure 4.10

Late-stage inflammation. Note the presence of lymphocytes, macrophages and giant cells.

Mediators of inflammation

The factors responsible for initiating the up-regulation of adhesion molecules on periductal vascular endothelial cells have not been identified; however, histological evidence is suggestive that pro-inflammatory cytokines may be involved. Ingham and co-workers studied the pro-inflammatory cytokine content of 108 acne comedones, since comedones may subsequently develop into inflamed lesions. The presence of interleukins IL-1α, IL-β and IL-6 plus tumour necrosis factor (TNF)-α were determined using both bioassays and ELISAs. Biologically active IL-1α was present at high levels in 76% of comedones, while the other cytokines were rare. Moreover, in 58% of comedones, the levels of biologically active IL-1α exceeded 100 pg/mg of comedone material. Other studies have shown that the injection of around 100 pg of IL-1α into the dermis of volunteers is sufficient to promote inflammation.

Thus in acne, the majority of comedones clearly represent a 'dermal pool' of pro-inflammatory IL-1α. Since spongiosis of the pilosebaceous follicle wall is a feature of early inflammatory change, this could lead to leakage of comedonal IL-1α into the dermis. The consequence would be activation of dermal microvascular endothelial cells, selective accumulation of antigen non-specific mononuclear cells and initiation of antigen independent cutaneous inflammation. The scenario is totally consistent with the histological features of early inflammation in acne. An amplification phase via antigen-dependent T-cell responses to other comedonal components, for example *Propionibacterium acnes*, might then develop. The intensity and duration of the subsequent cell-mediated response would depend on many factors, including the degree of individual sensitization to their cutaneous microflora. Following disruption of the follicle wall, neutrophils would be attracted

inflamed lesions. Although deep-seated lesions are more likely to result in acne scarring, some patients with papulopustular lesions have scarring.

The factors that contribute to scar formation have not been investigated. This is an important area for future research since scarring is of major concern to some patients whose acne has resolved.

into the duct by microbial chemotactic factors. Much work in the early 1980s in the USA by Puhvel and co-workers, and Leyden and co-workers demonstrated the capability of *P. acnes* to attract neutrophils in vitro. Data from both sides of the Atlantic has also demonstrated that complement activation is involved in the early to later stages of inflammation (Figure 4.11) and that *P. acnes* is capable of triggering both the alternative and classical complement pathways.

> • Certain cytokines, in particular IL-1α, may be a trigger to acne inflammation

The role of cutaneous micro-organisms in inflammatory acne cannot be overlooked. There is considerable evidence to suggest that *P. acnes* is important, since treatments that reduce the number of *P. acnes* organisms are therapeutically successful and the failure of antibiotic therapy in acne has been associated with the development of *P. acnes* resistance.

Whether *P. acnes* plays a role in the initiation of inflammation in acne is questionable since not all lesions are colonized (Table 4.2). Nevertheless, there is an increase in the

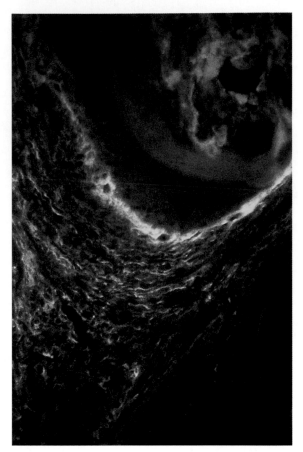

Figure 4.11

Deposition of complement (yellow-green colour) in the basement membrane of a microcomedone. This demonstrates that complement is also involved in the later stages of inflammation.

Table 4.2   The prevalence and population density of *P. acnes* colonizing acne lesions and normal follicles from the back.

	Prevalence (%)	Geometric mean colony forming units per colonized follicle
Normal follicles	17	8.0×10^4
Closed comedones	46	1.2×10^5
Open comedones	75	2.9×10^5
1-day-old papules	68	2.7×10^5
3-day-old papules	79	5.5×10^5

number of lesions colonized by *P. acnes* following early inflammatory change. *P. acnes* is a potent adjuvant that induces a chronic inflammatory tissue response because it is resistant to phagocyte killing and degradation. Patients with severe acne are significantly more sensitized to *P. acnes* than normal individuals, and the overall immunological status of patients is elevated compared with acne-free individuals of the same age. These observations do not provide direct evidence for a pathogenic role of *P. acnes* in initiating inflammatory acne and may merely reflect an increased exposure of patients to the organism as a result of their condition. However, it is inconceivable that colonization of inflamed lesions by this potent adjuvant does play a role in the exacerbation of the chronic inflammatory response.

- It is likely but not proven that *P. acnes* plays an important role in acne inflammation

---

Part II: Clinical features

5 Clinical features of acne

Introduction

Acne vulgaris is rarely, if ever, misdiagnosed by the dermatologist and so its clinical features should require very little explanation. The disorder is recognized by most lay people let alone the physician. Nevertheless, it is important to describe in reasonable detail the clinical features of acne, particularly since therapy may be dictated by lesion type. Although these topics have been discussed briefly in the introduction to this book, it is appropriate in this chapter to extend the introductory remarks.

Natural history of acne

The age of onset of acne is earlier in females because of their earlier onset of adolescence (Figure 5.1). Females develop acne usually around 12 or 13 years and males at around 13 or 14 years; on close examination, however, in a good light, it is common to see blackheads and whiteheads in 8- and 9-year-old boys and girls. Non-inflamed lesions are the first type of acne lesions, and inflammatory lesions occur later. Peak severity of acne is 17–18 years in females and 19–21 years in males.

Figure 5.1

The age of onset of acne in males and females.

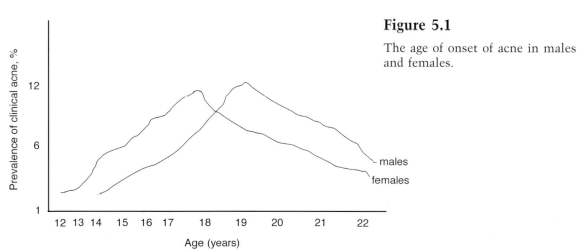

Detailed examination of the skin of most adolescents will reveal at least a few lesions; this is referred to as physiological acne. In many, the physiological acne will clear up within 3–4 years. Those with clinical acne and who require help from the physician, however, will have the disease for 8–12 years. In the majority of such individuals, the acne will have cleared by the age of 25 years. In 7%, however, the acne does persist well into the third and fourth decade and exceptionally into the fifth, sixth and seventh decade. There are a small group of individuals who develop late-onset acne, starting beyond the age of 25 years.

Acne is a polymorphous dermatosis with a polygenetic background. It does not follow Mendelian rules: however, if both parents had severe acne as adolescents, their children are likely to present with clinical acne in puberty. Studies of identical twins show that both twins are affected with acne in about 98% of all cases (Figure 5.2). In particular, the age of onset and the sebum excretion rate and number of comedones are very similar but, despite a similar age of onset the inflammatory severity of acne is not identical. This supports the concept that 'exogenous'

factors, such as colonization with *P. acnes*, modulate the inflammatory expression of acne. In contrast, in a study of heterozygotic twins, only one twin was affected in half the cases and there was little or no similarity in their sebum production and comedones (Figure 5.3). Not unexpectedly, there was no similarity in the number of inflammatory lesions.

There is, however, evidence that atopic individuals have a lower incidence of acne. The reason may in part be due to a lower sebum excretion and different sebum pattern. A special subtype of acne was recognized to be linked to an abnormal XYY-chromosome pattern. This XYY-pattern is found in 1 out of 1000 newborn. One out of seven with XYY-syndrome develop severe inflammatory acne of the conglobate type. Additional clinical features of these patients are a height of greater than 180 cm, some evidence of mental retardation and a tendency for aggressive behaviour. Whether this is part of the syndrome or a reaction to the severe and early development of conglobate acne is not known. Androgen levels and secretion are no different from those found in XY-conglobate acne patients.

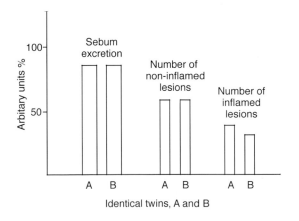

Figure 5.2

Types of lesions seen in identical twins.

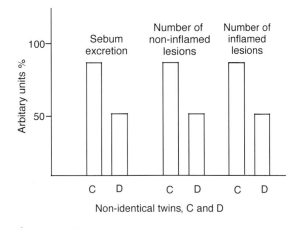

Figure 5.3

Types of lesions seen in non-identical twins.

Racial differences also exist. Caucasians are more prone to severe acne than black people; and both have more severe acne than Japanese. The racial difference in skin androgen effect is also reflected in other androgen-mediated cutaneous features. White Europeans and Americans may have androgenetic alopecia as well as fully and densely developed terminal hairs in the beard area, the opposite is true in Japanese.

- Age of onset of acne is typically 12–15 years
- Peak severity of acne is 17–21 years
- 93% of cases of acne are resolved by 25 years
- Acne persists in 7% up to the age of 45 years
- Genetic factors may be important in the aetiology of acne

Importance of the menstrual cycle in acne

Of female acne patients, 70% report a deterioration of the disease during the premenstrual days of their cycle. Most female acne patients have a regular cycle and many have normal levels of circulating hormones. Certain hormones such as androgens have a pro-inflammatory action, and so variation in androgens or their modification by anti-androgens could influence the inflammatory severity. A further explanation for the premenstrual flare could be a variation in sebaceous pore size. Direct in vivo microscopy demonstrated that the orifice of the pilosebaceous duct was smallest between Days 16–20 of the menstrual cycle. This could reduce sebum flow and so increase the possibility of inflammatory mediators to concentrate in the lumen of the duct, thus stimulating a flare of acne premenstrually.

Are acne patients hormonal misfits?

As explained in Part I of this book, most patients with acne have normal hormone levels or levels at the upper end of the normal range. Acne patients are not endocrine misfits. Neither do they usually suffer from abnormal irregular periods, excess hair and nor do they have androgenetic alopecia. They have no problems in mixing with the opposite sex apart from psychological stress that may impair such relationships. In later years, conception and pregnancy are not usually a problem in subjects with acne. Thus, clinically, this data confirms a long-held impression that most acne patients are not hormonal misfits. There is usually no need whatsoever to investigate a female patient for hormonal problems.

Some exceptional cases warrant investigation; namely children who develop acne between 3–7 years, individuals who have responded poorly to treatment (e.g. the patient who had required three courses of oral isotretinoin and/or who has other skin androgenic features such as excessive hair and female-pattern alopecia). If appropriate, such patients should be examined fully to detect any clinical clues as to the underlying endocrinopathy causing the acne. Investigations will focus on ovarian, adrenal and pituitary causes of excessive androgen production. Particular reference should be given to the possibility of polycystic ovarian syndrome and late-onset congenital adrenal hyperplasia. Investigations could include the following:

- Total plasma testosterone and free testosterone)
- Sex hormone binding globulin (SHBG)
- Dihydroepiandrostencdione (DHEA)
- Follicule stimulating hormone (FSH)
- Luteinising hormone (LH)
- Prolactin

Figure 5.4

(a) Ultrasound scan of the ovaries in a patient with polycystic ovarian syndrome. (b) A diagnostic work-up for endocrinological investigation of a patient suspected of excess androgen production.

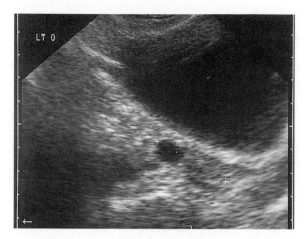

(a)

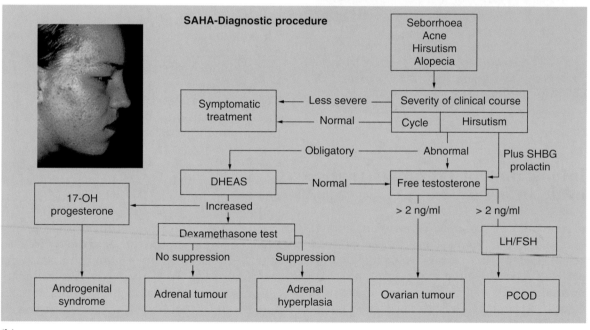

(b)

If the clinician suspects late-onset adrenal hyperplasia, it is necessary to take a blood sample at 9.00 am for 17α-hydroxyprogesterone. If the latter level is raised, further investigation should be performed, including a dexamethasone test. Other investigations may include an ultrasound of the ovaries to detect anatomically polycystic ovaries (Figure 5.4). In this situation better results are obtained with a transvaginal ultrasound rather than an abdominal ultrasound investigation, if deemed appropriate.

- Most acne patients are not hormonal misfits
- Occasionally it is necessary to exclude polycystic ovarian syndrome and late-onset congenital adrenal hyperplasia

A certain type of female patient expresses several symptoms of androgen-related target cell type function or peripheral increased androgen metabolism. These patients have seborrhoea, acne, hirsutism and alopecia, SAHA-syndrome. Here a careful endocrinological examination is important.

SAHA syndrome is a familial, ovarian, adrenal, pituitary and endocrine disorder. The combination of SAHA plus acanthosis nigricans was named HAIR-AN syndrome. It is important to note that patients with SAHA syndrome need a careful endocrinological examination (Figure 5.4b). Furthermore, in patients showing hyperandrogenism and polycystic ovaries, insulin resistance has to be excluded.

Does diet influence acne?

Many years ago, the importance of diet was overestimated. Chocolates, caramels and fatty foods were accused of aggravating acne. A double-blind controlled study demonstrated that a diet high in chocolate did not modulate the natural course of acne. In a more detailed study, no correlation could be found between acne severity and food ingestion, whatever the diet.

Nevertheless, continuous low-caloric intake such as in patients with anorexia nervosa may improve the disease. Such dietary fads and crash-diets are capable of reducing the sebum excretion rate and may change the composition of sebum. These diets decrease sex hormones such as DHEA, which may also explain the clinical improvement seen. However, crash diets combined with strong physical stress can increase androgen release.

> • Overall dietary factors do not cause acne

Ultraviolet light and acne

There is little scientific data on the inter-relationships between ultraviolet (UV) radiation and acne. Tanning of the skin produces a camouflage that leads to a subjective improvement of acne. Erythematous and suberythematous doses of UVB can lead to scaling of the interfollicular epidermis and may help desquamate corneocytes from around the acroinfundibulum. UV radiation helps many skin diseases. Narrow band UVB particularly helps in eczema and psoriasis. Although UV radiation is known to have a wide-ranging effect on cellular immunological systems, controlled studies on the therapeutic effects are lacking. Nevertheless, it has been demonstrated in animal experiments that UVA can convert squalene into squalene peroxide, which may enhance rather than reduce comedogenesis. *P. acnes* produces porphyrins. Recently, it has been shown that wavelengths between 400–450 nm can activate porphyrins in the bacteria and help destroy *P. acnes* in the acne follicle. Visible light in both the red and blue light range has been shown to improve acne as effectively as benzoyl peroxide; it is suggested that the red light (wavelength × nm) is antimicrobial. Photodynamic therapies are currently under investigation.

> • Natural sunlight and visible light are beneficial to acne
> • How UV radiation improves acne is unknown

Humidity

It is known from clinical observations that acne can worsen dramatically if patients are exposed to tropical and subtropical climates. Severe outbreaks of acne were observed among French, British and American soldiers in Vietnam, Korea and Malaysia. Holidays in

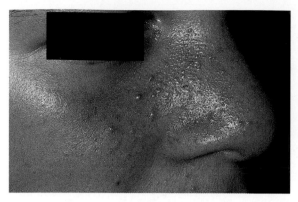

Figure 5.5

Acne Mallorca. This patient had virtually no acne when she went on holiday, but within 2 weeks of a hot, sweaty holiday in Mallorca, developed what is clinically called 'acne Mallorca'. This is typified by sudden onset of relatively monomorphic papular pustular lesions.

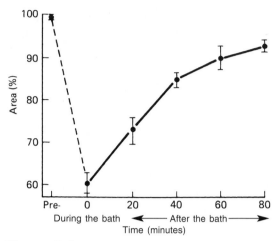

Figure 5.6

Hydration of the skin associated with reduction in the size of the sebaceous follicular pore. This graph shows percentage area of pore size with time before during and after a hot bath.

humid environments frequently precipitate acne, contributing to the clinical picture of the so-called 'Acne Mallorca' (Figure 5.5); moreover, holidays in Southern Europe often produce an acne flare. The reason for humid environments precipitating acne is not well investigated but may relate to an increased poral occlusive effect of skin hydration. Direct in vivo microscopy has confirmed such changes (Figure 5.6). Besides heat and humidity, friction might contribute to additional acne by irritating the upper parts of the pilosebaceous duct.

- Excess humidity aggravates acne by an effect on sebum outflow

---

Acne-associated symptoms

It is usually the change in physical appearance that brings the patient to the physician, but in a few patients there are complaints of pain and itching. Inflammatory acne and acne scarring cause many psychosocial problems, particularly since it develops and persists in the rather sensitive adolescent acne years. The disease can cause loss of self-esteem, loss of confidence, obsessive traits, anxiety and depression. Several quality-of-life studies have shown that acne patients may have difficulties in coping with life and may even have employment problems as a result of the acne. One study has shown acne to be associated with suicidal ideation in up to 5% of acne outpatients. Some patients are pleased with the outcome of therapy on their inflamed lesions but remain equally affected psychosocially because of resultant scarring.

Although itching is an uncommon symptom it may occur particularly in the early and successful phases of treatment. It is suggested that the itch may result from the release of histamine-like compounds released from *P. acnes*, which have been killed as a consequence of therapy.

Low-grade pain is also unusual but is a major feature of patients who have nodules and sinus tracts, especially on the trunk. Such patients may also complain of the unsightliness that occurs as a result of the bleeding crusty lesions.

Examination of the skin

It is necessary to examine the skin using good and constant lighting, both in terms of overhead and focused light. The authors prefer to use a Brighton 1001. It is important to move the light and the patient's skin at different angles, otherwise the physician may miss many whiteheads, leading to inappropriate topical therapy. It is also necessary to stretch the skin to avoid overlooking the presence of non-inflamed lesions.

In the clinic it is essential to grade the acne severity. The authors would like to recommend a new pictorial grading scale, which was published in the *Journal of Dermatological Treatment* (1998) **9**: 215–220.

It is almost virtually impossible for the physician or even the patient to remember just what the acne looked like at the previous visit compared with the current visit. The authors therefore strongly recommend the use of reference photographs for the face (Figure 5.7), for the back (Figure 5.8) and for the chest (Figure 5.9). Such reference pictures are essential for the optimum management of the acne patient.

It is also necessary to assess the lesion type. There are fundamentally three types of lesions:

- Non-inflamed lesions
- Inflamed lesions
- Scarring

Non-inflamed lesions

Five types of non-inflamed lesions exist:

- Microcomedones
- Blackheads
- Whiteheads
- Macrocomedones (microcysts)
- Miscellaneous comedones

Microcomedone

This is a histological diagnosis (Figure 5.10). If a biopsy is taken of the 'normal' looking skin of a patient's back with acne, in 27% of cases one will biopsy a microcomedone, which frequently is the forerunner of an inflamed lesion or another non-inflamed lesion.

Blackheads

Blackheads really need no description (Figure 5.11). Suffice to say that the black of the blackhead is probably caused by oxidation of melanin but there may be other reasons.

Whiteheads

Contrary to much clinical expectation, whiteheads, when examined for appropriately, are much more frequent than black heads. They are macular or papular lesions 0.5–3.0 mm in diameter, but most are 1 mm or less (Figure 5.12). Although often quite difficult to see, with experience they are easily recognized.

Macrocomedones

Macrocomedones (microcysts) are usually whiteheads but occasionally blackheads that are over 3 mm (usually 3–5 mm) in diameter (Figure 5.13). Such lesions are frequently the focus of cosmetic problems, and sometimes the focus of inflammatory

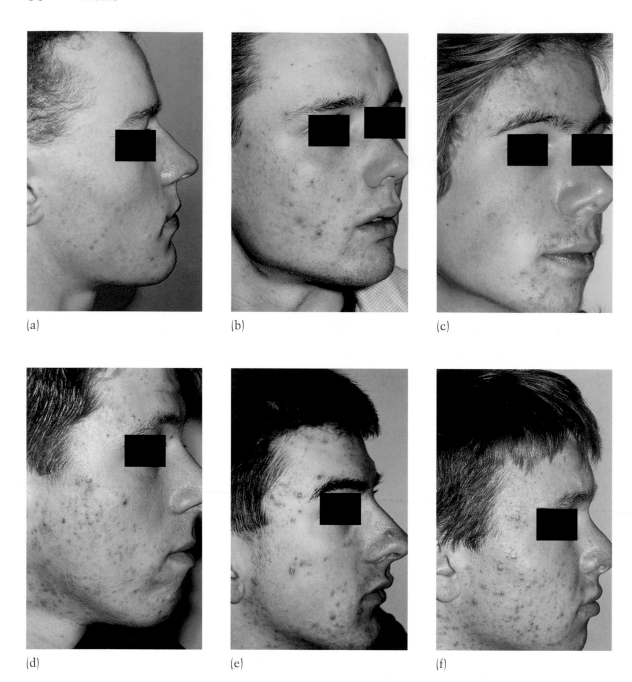

(a)   (b)   (c)

(d)   (e)   (f)

Figure 5.7

Grades of facial acne. (a) Grade 1; (b) Grade 2; (c) Grade 3; (d) Grade 4; (e) Grade 5; (f) Grade 6;
(g) Grade 7; (h) Grade 8; (i) Grade 9; (j) Grade 10; (k) Grade 11; (l) Grade 12.

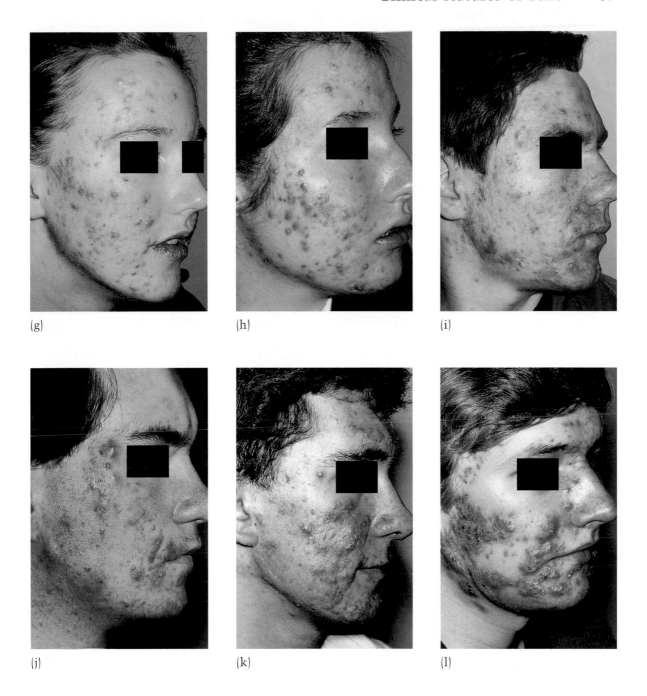

(g)

(h)

(i)

(j)

(k)

(l)

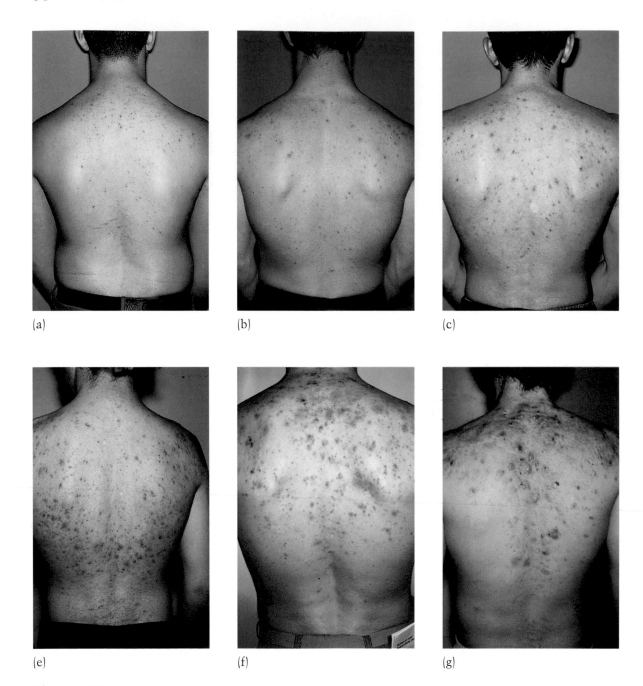

Figure 5.8

Grades of acne on the back. (a) Grade 1; (b) Grade 2; (c) Grade 3; (d) Grade 4; (e) Grade 5; (f) Grade 6; (g) Grade 7; (h) Grade 8.

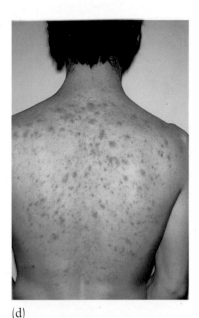

(d)

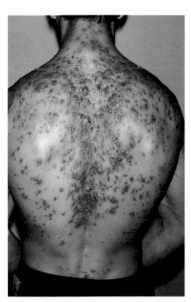

(h)

flares especially if patients are prescribed oral isotretinoin. They are often located at the upper lateral cheeks and pre- and post-articular areas.

Miscellaneous comedones

Types of comedones other than microcomedones, blackheads, whiteheads and macrocomedones also exist.

Sandpaper comedones are multiple, small, closely packed whiteheads that give the skin a rough sandpaper feel (Figure 5.14). Patients with this type of acne eventually usually require oral isotretinoin therapy. Recently, a clinical subtype with right blindness and keratosis follicularis with a retinol binding protein deficiency was described.

Submarine comedones are large, (5–8 mm in diameter) (Figures 5.15 and 5.16) and are often the focus of repeated inflamed lesions. Unless these comedones are treated by focal general cautery then the repetitive inflamed lesions persist (Figure 5.17).

• Pomade or cosmetic acne is induced by certain cosmetics or pomades, the latter being used to 'de-friz' the hair in Afro-Caribbeans (Figure 5.18). These comedones typically present as remarkably similarly sized whiteheads at the affected sites.

Inflammatory lesions

Inflammatory lesions are either superficial or deep.

Superficial acne lesions

These may either be papules (Figure 5.19) or pustules (Figure 5.20). Such lesions are less

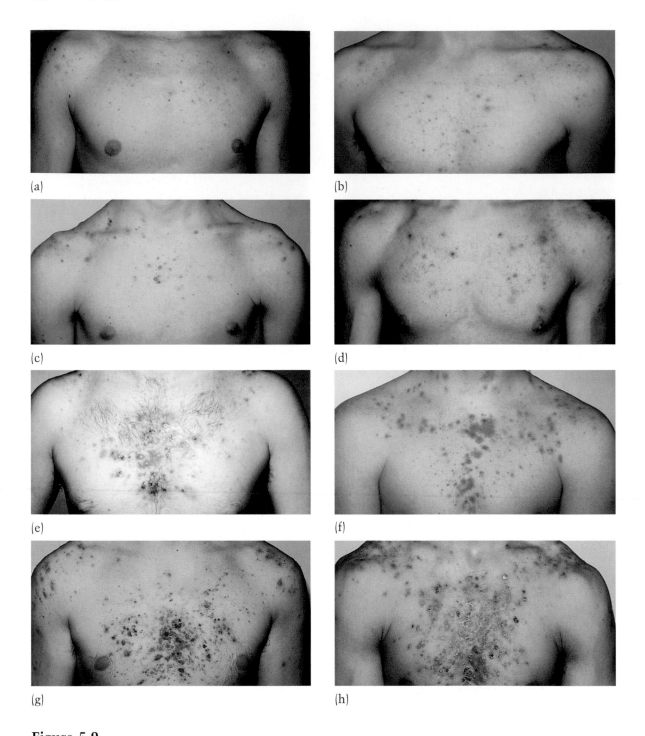

Figure 5.9

Grades of acne on the chest. (a) Grade 1; (b) Grade 2; (c) Grade 3; (d) Grade 4; (e) Grade 5; (f) Grade 6; (g) Grade 7; (h) Grade 8.

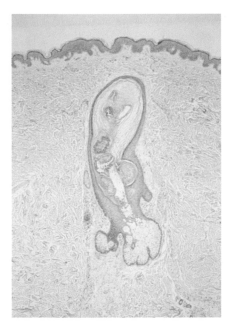

Figure 5.10

Histology of an early acne lesion. This microcomedone was not clinically evident.

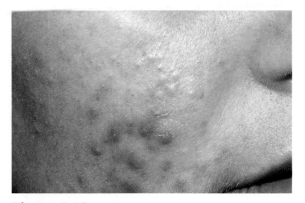

Figure 5.12

In the upper cheek there are some typical whiteheads. In the lower cheek there is a group of actively inflamed papules, two or three of which show early pustule formation.

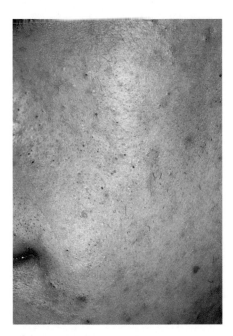

Figure 5.11

Typical blackheads.

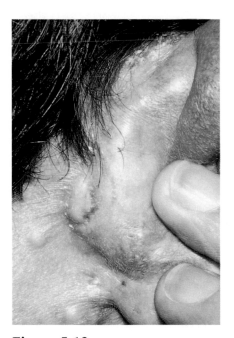

Figure 5.13

Macrocomedones which are usually closed comedones, occasionally open comedones, greater than 1 mm in diameter.

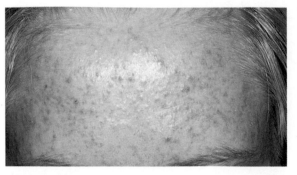

Figure 5.14

Patient with sandpaper comedone acne. Multiple small closely packed whiteheads give the skin a rough sandpaper feel.

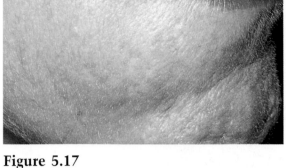

Figure 5.17

The same patient as in Figure 5.15/5.16, after gentle cautery to several areas of submarine comedones. This treatment resulted in resolution of the inflammatory lesions.

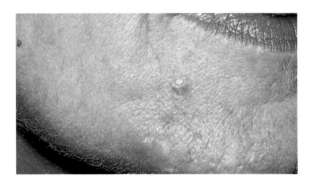

Figure 5.15

This patient had persistent inflammatory nodules.

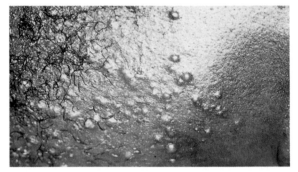

Figure 5.18

Afro-Caribbean patient with typical pomade acne. Multiple similar looking whiteheads are present.

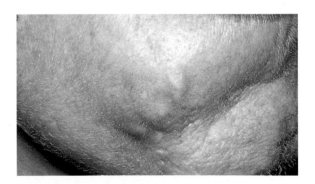

Figure 5.16

Examination of submarine comedones. On stretching of the skin it is possible to see the underlying large submarine comedones.

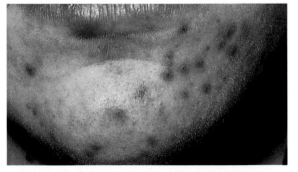

Figure 5.19

A patient with actively inflamed papules.

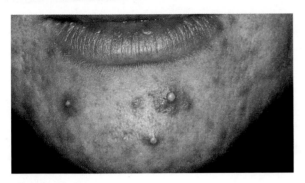

Figure 5.20

A different patient to that shown in Figure 5.19, showing many pustules.

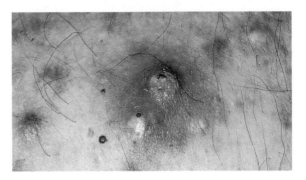

Figure 5.22

Patient with large pustules.

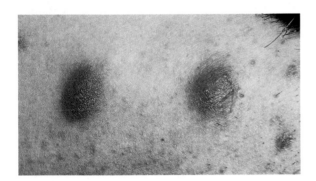

Figure 5.21

Acne nodules.

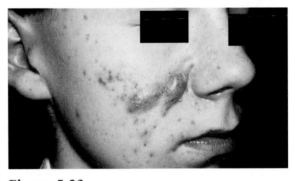

Figure 5.23

Inflammatory sinus tract that might respond a little to potent topical steroids.

than 1 cm in diameter (usually 1–3 mm) and are either red or pus-filled depending on whether it is a papule or pustule. Such lesions can also be described as active if redder, more yellow and larger (more pus-filled) than less active lesions. Many combinations of lesions such as papular/pustular lesions and the like may be described; however, the authors consider that there is no clinical benefit in having many hybrid descriptions. The physician should appreciate that many lesions can show several features of the basic inflamed lesions, namely papules and pustules.

Deep inflammatory lesions

Deeper inflammatory lesions may be either nodules (Figure 5.21) or deep pustules (Figure 5.22). Nodules can be classed as small nodules if 5–10 mm and large nodules if greater than 1 cm. Such nodules can even be up to 2–3 cm in diameter. Nodules are initially firm, tender and very red. Over time, nodules become softer and the overlying skin may break, producing a haemorrhagic crust, which is very unsightly. Deep pustules are softer, 1 cm or more in size, they may arise from a nodule but can arise de novo from a small inflammatory pustule. The lesion often ruptures much earlier than a nodule and may also produce haemorrhagic crusting.

Extensions of such deep lesions are what are referred to as sinus tracks (Figure 5.23). Such lesions are often dumb-bell shaped and frequently consist of two nodules that have been joined together by a subepithelial structure which is a focus of continuous and intermittent inflammation. Such lesions are very difficult to treat and are characterized by recurrence and cause much anguish for the patient and physician. These lesions inevitably scar.

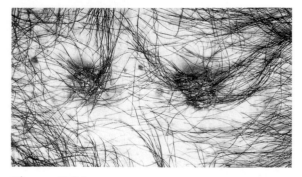

Figure 5.24

Site of two deep inflammatory lesions.

Haemorrhagic crusts

Some of the larger deeper lesions may occasionally go through the phase of haemorrhagic crusting (Figure 5.24).

Macular formation

Very early inflammatory lesions are often recognized as transient slightly pink macules. Such lesions develop relatively quickly into a papule or pustule. Macules also occur as the late stage of the resolving papule/pustule or nodule (Figures 5.25 and 5.26). These late stage macules are usually on close examination associated with a little scaling.

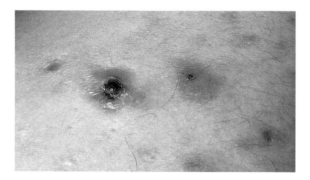

Figure 5.25

Macules. This usually represents the late stage of resolving inflammatory lesions.

Scarring

There are fundamentally two sorts of scarring: (i) where there is loss of scar tissue (e.g. ice-pick scars, atrophic macular scars and perifollicular elastolysis) and (ii) where there is an increase of collagen tissue (e.g. keloid and hypertrophic scars). Although patients with severe inflammatory acne scar, a significant number of patients who scar

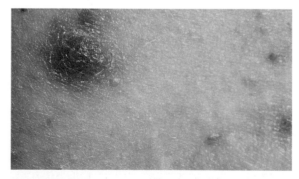

Figure 5.26

The lesion on the left was a nodule 2 weeks prior to taking the picture. On the day the picture was taken, the large lesion could not be palpated. It was a macule.

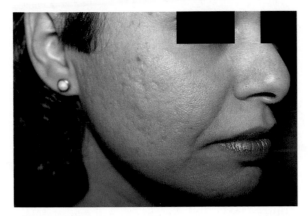

Figure 5.27

Typical ice-pick scar. These deep, jagged scars have a well-defined edge.

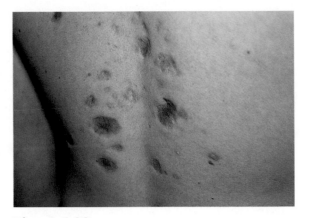

Figure 5.28

The early phases of atrophic macular scars are typically red or violaceous in colour and may, as shown here, be depressed below the surface of the normal skin.

have never had such extensive and deep-nodular acne. They simply have the common papular and pustular varieties of acne, which can scar in many patients. Early evidence suggests that the potential for scarring runs in families; this remains to be proven.

Ice-pick scars

Ice-picks scars (Figure 5.27) typically occur on the cheeks and consist of small, superficial to deep jagged scars, the edge of which are usually very well defined and at right angles to the skin surface. The base of the scar may be extendable, but sometimes there is a white fibrotic base where the scar is tethered to the underlying tissue.

Atrophic macular scars

Atrophic macular scars are lesions that are usually 5–20 mm in size. The surface is soft and initially red. They become much more inflamed in situations of increased body temperature, such as exercise and increased room temperature (Figure 5.28). With time,

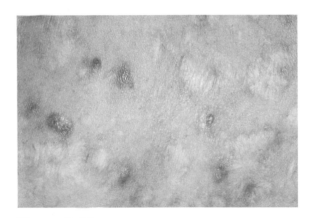

Figure 5.29

In time, atrophic macular scars become much paler and as seen here are white in colour and have a wrinkly surface.

Figure 5.30

Perifollicular elastolysis is difficult to photograph but this patient had many such lesions. Typically, they are macular lesions although occasionally they are just palpable. To the uninitiated, they look not unlike a whitehead and may possibly represent aborted comedones, but the precise aetiology is unknown. As the name suggests, histologically there is loss of elastic tissue.

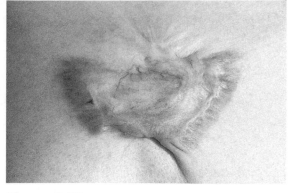

Figure 5.32

A keloid scar. This is a firm scar that has extended beyond the site of original inflammation.

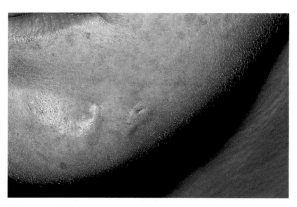

Figure 5.31

A firm hypertrophic scar. This type of scar does not extend beyond the site of original inflammation.

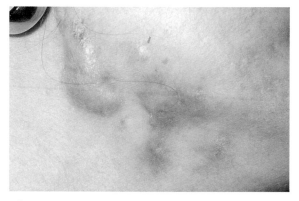

Figure 5.33

A keloid scar that has become paler with age.

over a period of months, they change to a violet colour and eventually to pale lilac or white (Figure 5.29). Although such scars are soft, there is sometimes an element of deeper fibrosis making the scar adhere to the under-lying tissues.

Perifollicular elastolysis

Perifollicular elastolysis (PFE) predominantly occurs on the back, chest and neck (Figure 5.30). It has been speculated that lesions may arise from whiteheads that have aborted and not developed into inflamed lesions. It is suggested that, as a result of an elastase enzyme produced by *P. acnes* there is loss of elastic tissue around the follicle producing lesions, that are similar to whiteheads, but with a softer and slightly irregular surface. With experience it is not too difficult to distinguish one from the other. PFE are persistent, whereas whiteheads will eventually develop into inflamed lesions and resolve either spontaneously or with therapy.

Hypertrophic scars

Hypertrophic scars, as with keloid scars, represent the presence of excessive fibrous tissue with marked vascularization.

Hypertrophic scars are moderately firm or firm papules or nodules that are the same size as the initiating inflammatory lesion (Figure 5.31). The skin surface is smooth and pink.

Keloid scars

The physical signs of keloids are similar to those associated with hypertrophic scars, except that the scars have extended beyond the dimensions of the original inflammatory lesion and are less vascularized (Figure 5.32). Consequently, keloids tend to be more irregular in shape and probably have less tendency to resolve spontaneously; however, some become paler in appearance (Figure 5.33).

6 Differential diagnosis

Acne usually poses no diagnostic difficulties for the clinician. Occasionally, however, there is ambiguity. This chapter gives a guide to the differential diagnosis. The diseases described below are the most important ones and are listed in alphabetical order and not in order of frequency or occurrence.

Tables 6.1–6.4 may help the physician in separating acne mimics from acne itself.

Table 6.1 Acneiform dermatoses mimic acne vulgaris or other subtypes

Differences
  Other than common localization
  Independent of age
  Sudden onset
  Monomorphic, mostly follicular bound
  Later comedone development
  Exogenous trigger or inducer

Table 6.2 Main provoking agents of acneiform dermatoses

Corticosteroids	Anticonvulsives
IHN	Antidepressants
Vitamins $B_{1,6,12}$, D (?)	Lithium
Halogens	Amineptin
Iodide	Disulfiram
Bromide	Chinin
Cyclosporin	Azathioprin
Thiouracil	Phenobarbiturate
Tetracyclines	PUVA, UVA
	X-ray (cobalt)

Table 6.3 Differences between typical acne and acneiform dermatoses

	Acne vulgaris	Acneiform dermatoses
Localization	Sebaceous gland follicle	All follicle types
Distribution	Face, trunk	All areas
Etiology	Target cell hyperresponsiveness to androgens P. acnes, immunoresponse	Drugs; diet factors; infections; UVA
Primary lesion	Comedone	Papule, pustule
Secondary lesion	Papule, pustule	Comedone

Table 6.4   Differences between typical acne and acneiform dermatoses

	Acne vulgaris	*Acneiform dermatoses*
Clinically	Polymorphous	Monomorphous
Scarring	Yes	Minimal
Onset	Slowly around puberty	Suddenly, every age group
Course	Regressing ~20 years or prolonged	Depending on provoking agent

Acne agminata

Acne agminata is a very uncommon condition presenting with acne-like lesions on the face (Figure 6.1). Unless the patient has co-existing acne, however, there are no comedones. Lesions all look remarkably similar, being small, brown or red granulomatous acniform papules. The lesions are often closely packed and symmetrically distributed suborbitally on the cheeks and chin, although they usually resolve spontaneously after 2 or 3 years, they frequently leave scars of the atrophic macular variety. Treatment is difficult: options include oral dapsone, lamprene and oral isotretinoin – dapsone and lamprene are probably the most beneficial agents. In skin types IV–VI the erbium YAG-laser can be tried.

Acne varioliformis

This is a condition that appears to be seen less frequently than it was some 20–30 years ago. It typically occurs in females between the ages of 30–60 years. Frequently, it is difficult to find a primary lesion: the physician usually sees an excoriated papule (Figure 6.2), since rarely is a presenting papule or pustule detected. The lesions may be seen on the face and especially on the upper trunk. The characteristic feature of this disease is that they leave a varioliform (i.e. smallpox-like) scar, hence the name. The aetiology is unknown, but this needs to be distinguished from nodular prurigo in atopic individuals as well as from acne. In some patients acne

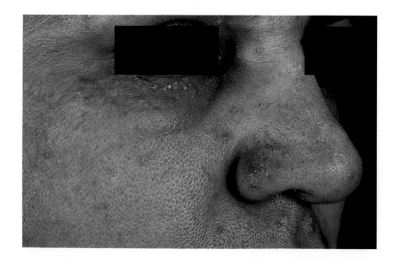

Figure 6.1

Patient with localized form of acne agminata.

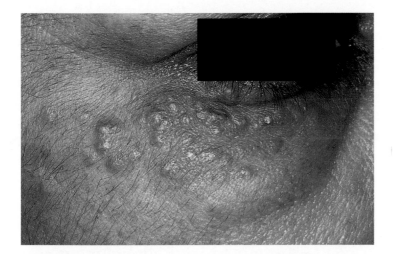

Figure 6.2

Close-up view of lesions in a patient with acne agminata.

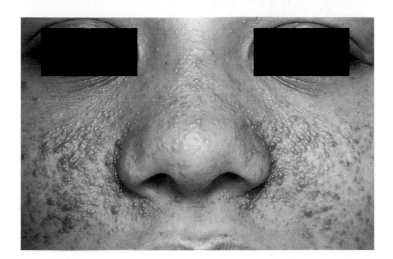

Figure 6.3

The fleshy red lesions of adenoma sebaceum.

lesions and prurigo papules of atopic dermatitis may coexist raising therapeutic problems. Some physicians consider it to be a variant of dermatitis artefacta. Treatment is very unsatisfactory and varied. Steroid-antibiotic combinations, such as momethasone cream combined with an antiseptic may help, along with systemic antibiotics and oral antihistamines. Topical antimicrobials such as pseudomonic acid may be worth a try.

Adenoma sebaceum

This condition presents in early adolescence with fleshy, red lesions on the forehead and cheeks, which are especially prominent around the nose. Adenoma sebaceum is a misnomer, because histologically it is characterized by angiofibromas and trichoepitheliomas. Occasionally such lesions develop earlier in life and become more prominent at puberty (Figure 6.3). The patient will have other features of the disease, such as a shagreen patch over the sacrum, periungual fibromas, epilepsy and mental retardation (Bournville–Pringle disease). Confusion usually arises if adenoma sebaceum co-exists with acne.

Boils

These are rarely confused with acne. The patient presents with a nodular or deep pustular lesion or lesions. The lesions that develop over a few days are tender and usually burst within a few days. If the lesions are multiple, there may be a systemic reaction in the form of a fever. A swab will demonstrate the presence of *Staphylococcus aureus*. The patient responds well to appropriate anti-staphylococcal therapy, for example flucloxacillin.

Dental sinus

This normally only constitutes a problem if co-existent with acne. Typically a patient with average acne responds well except for a persistent large nodule (Figure 6.4a), which is usually located on the chin. A radiograph of the teeth will demonstrate dental caries and a sinus tract from the apex of the tooth to the skin (Figure 6.4b). Removal of the tooth is required.

Human immunodeficiency virus (HIV)

Patients with HIV may present with a variety of acneform rashes, including eosinophilic folliculitis (Figure 6.5). The patients have widespread papular eruptions,

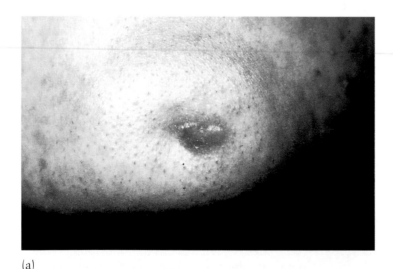

(a)

Figure 6.4

Dental sinus. (a) This patient had acne that responded well to treatment but was left with a persistent nodule. (b) This nodule was a dental sinus confirmed by radiography.

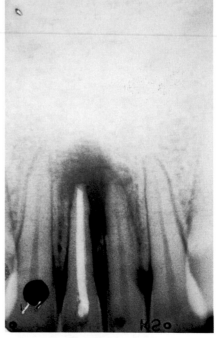

(b)

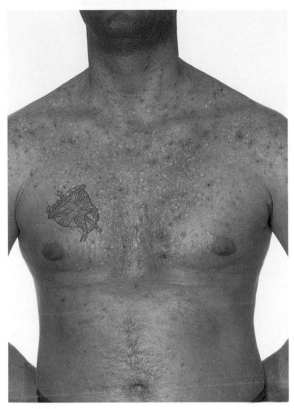

Figure 6.5

Patient with an acneform rash that is typical of eosinophilic folliculitis in a patient with HIV.

no non-inflammatory lesions and often the lesions occur both inside and outside the acne-prone area.

Folliculitis

Several types of folliculitis may masquerade as acne:

S. aureus *folliculitis*

Folliculitis caused by colonization with *Staphylococcus aureus* on the face can

sometimes be misdiagnosed as acne. The prominent lesions are superficial follicular pustules that are often distributed on the lateral cheeks, the chin and the temporal site of the forehead. Such lesions are usually of relatively sudden onset. Such patients are best treated with oral antibiotics such as flucoxacillin (250 mg qds for 5 days).

S. epidermis *folliculitis*

The folliculitis is caused by a superficial inflammation of the upper terminal and vellus hair follicle with *Staphylococcus epidermis*. The lesions are usually seen in men but can occur in the more hairy female. Lesions are chronic and particularly seen on the beard area, especially the neck, presenting as papules or superficial pustules. It is often referred to as a shaving rash. Treatment is difficult since *S. epidermis* is a skin commensal.

Antiseptic washes such as those containing Hibitane® and Polvidine® iodine may help. A change in shaving habit may occasionally help. Oral antibiotics, such as a 5-day course of flucoxacillin (250 mg qds) is sometimes tried, with a very variable and usually poor outcome.

Demodex folliculitis

Rarely, the folliculitis may be caused by demodex. Some clinicians deny the existence of demodex folliculitis. Demodex folliculitis (DF) occurs after overgrowth of this sapro-phyte in the follicles of the face. Mostly, it is located in the non-terminal hair-bearing areas of the skin, the forehead, nose and the cheeks (Figure 6.6a and b). The age of manifestation is usually the fifth to eighth decades of life. Enlarged follicular canals seem to be a predisposing factor. The typical

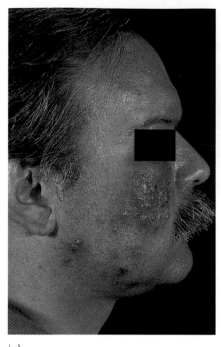

(a)

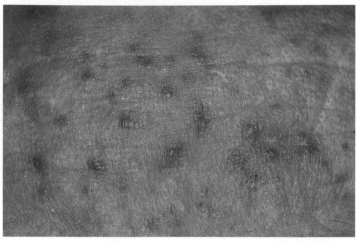

(b)

Figure 6.6

A patient with (a) a deeper located granulomatous demodex folliculitis and (b) a more papular–pustular acne-like type.

lesions are papulopustules, sometimes becoming confluent to form small plaques. A typical complication can be superinfection by staphylococci. Disruption of follicles may lead to granulomatous reactions. Lesions near to the lower eyelids can provoke demodex blepharitis. Topical application of lindane, 2% metronidazole or two cycles of systemic metronidazole for 5 days with a 2-week interval leads almost to a complete resolution of clinical lesions. Topical crotamiton or pyrethroids are alternatives.

Fungal folliculitis

A rare type of folliculitis is that caused by the yeast *Candida* or a tinea organism. The clinical presentation is similar to *S. epider-* *mis* folliculitis but it is more often an asymmetrical facial eruption and frequently occurs in younger patients. If *Candida* is isolated (Figure 6.7) therapy is with ketoconazole washing solution; if located more deeply in follicles, then orally with itraconazole; if a tinea organism is identified, then terbinafine therapy may be helpful.

Pityrosporum folliculitis

This was originally described as an acne-like eruption found particularly on the upper trunk. In contrast to acne, it is usually mildly itchy, consisting of papules and occasionally superficial pustules on an ill-defined erythematous background (Figure 6.8).

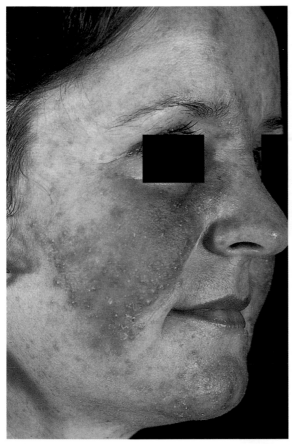

Figure 6.7

Patient with candida folliculitis in a pre-existing rosacea.

Milia

It is very rare for milia to be confused with acne by the experienced practitioner (Figure 6.9). Patients present with small, white or slightly yellow lesions, found especially on the eyelids or in the infraorbital area. Milia do not develop into inflamed lesions, rather they represent retention of cornified material in the duct of the sweat glands. Patients often find that they can gently squeeze out the material themselves. This can be performed in the clinic and is also performed by beauty

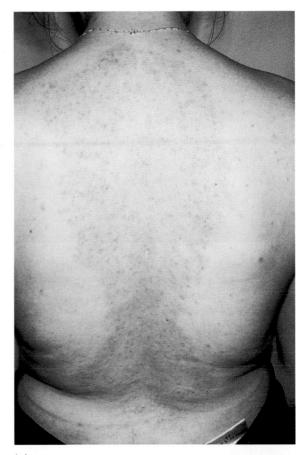

(a)

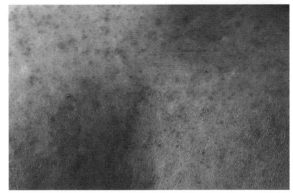

(b)

Figure 6.8

(a) Patient with ill-defined erythematous papular pustular lesions of pityrosporum folliculitis.
(b) Close-up of same patient.

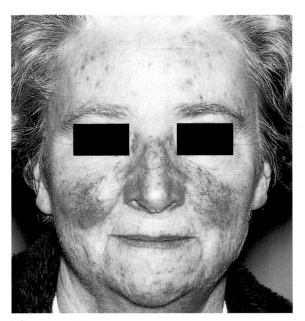

Figure 6.11

See below.

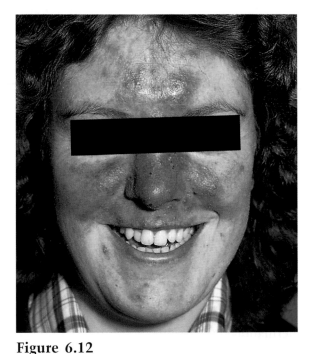

Figure 6.12

Two patients with typical rosacea showing typical redness, papules and pustules and some nodules (Figures 6.11 and 6.12).

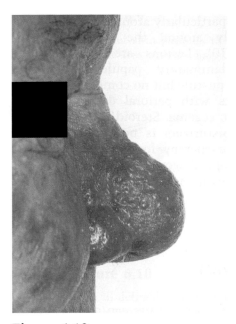

Figure 6.13

Typical rhinophyma grade II showing diffuse thickening of the nose associated with diffuse sebaceous hyperplasia.

Seborrhoeic dermatitis

In rare cases, a patient is referred who has no acne but has seborrhoeic dermatitis (Figure 6.15). Such a patient has a dry skin with erythematous scaly papules, particularly in the nasolabial folds and forehead. Frequently there is a family or personal history of asthma, eczema or hayfever (some may present with minor lesions of psoriasis) and similar lesions may be present in the upper chest, upper back, axilla, groin and scalp. Overgrowth of *P. ovale* is common. Comedonal lesions, however, are not present. Therapy consists of ketoconazole topically and of the occasional use of topical steroids, but moisturizers, medicated bath oils and sedating antihistamines are often prescribed. HIV infection should be ruled out.

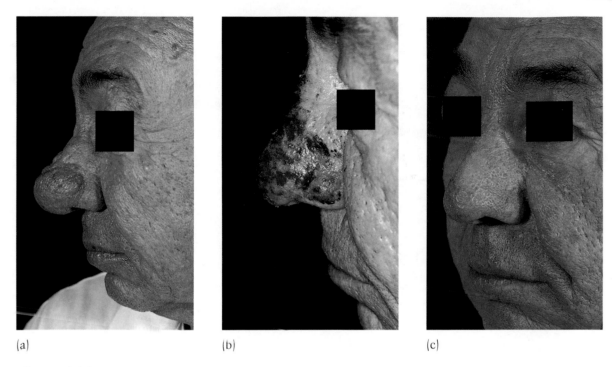

(a)   (b)   (c)

Figure 6.14

Rhinophyma grade II. (a) Before treatment; (b) part-way through treatment with a CO_2-laser; (c) at the end of treatment.

Sycosis barbae

This is not an uncommon disease especially in Afro-Caribbeans. In such individuals, there is a tendency for their hairs to curl even before they leave the hair canal. Consequently, they penetrate the upper part of the hair canal evoking a significant inflammatory reaction. Clinically, this presents as red/brown papules-pustules in the beard area, which are typified by chronicity and at times by hypertrophic scar formation (Figure 6.16).

Therapy is very difficult. A change in shaving habits may occasionally help; growing a beard may also help – it will certainly help to disguise some of the persistent papules. Oral and topical antibiotics, topical steroids and oral isotretinoin are of virtually no help.

Syringomas

These are frequently located at the suborbital area, slowly growing and mostly occurring in females. A special type is the disseminated one, almost located at the upper trunk. Electrocauterization, cryotherapy, CO_2-laser therapy or erbium YAG-laser are indicated (Figure 6.17).

Trichoepitheliomata

This uncommon disorder presents in the second and third decade as symmetrical flesh-coloured papules, typically in the perinasal and/or infraorbital areas (Figure 6.18).

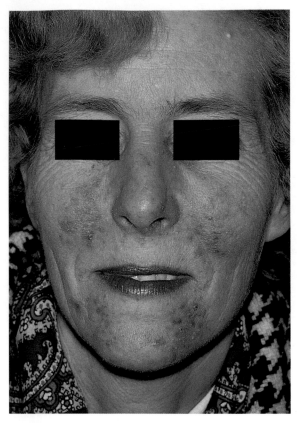

Figure 6.15

Patient with rosacea and seborrhoeic dermatitis. Ill-defined erythema and scaling are present.

SAPHO-Syndrome

SAPHO-(synovitis, acne, pustulosis, hyperostosis and osteitis) is an acronym that describes seronegative arthritis with preferential localization at the sterno-clavicular articulation. The dermatological manifestation are variable and include palmoplantar pustulosis, acne conglobata and fulminans, hidradenitis suppurativa or dissecting cellulitis of the scalp.

Differential acne scarring

Facial and trunkal scarring, thought to be caused by acne, is very rare and not caused by the acne. In some patients this so-called acne scarring is caused by other disorders, thus detailed history and clinical examination is necessary to detect other signs
Conditions implicated are:

- Hydroavacciniforme
- Ulerythema ophryogenes
- Atrophia maculosa varioliformis cutis (Figure 6.19)
- Porphyria cutanea tarda

The reader is referred to specialist texts for further information.

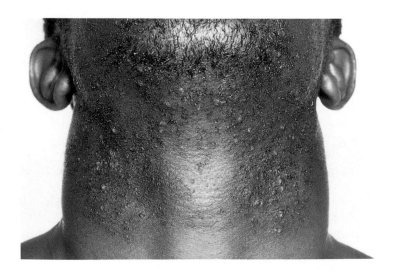

Figure 6.16

Sycosis barbae. In the beard earlier papules are often pigmented. Inflammation although present is often difficult to detect.

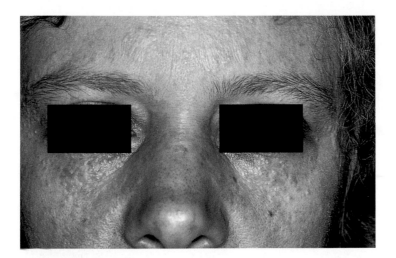

Figure 6.17

Syringomas – shows typical fleshy coloured lesions more typically seen in the infraorbital area.

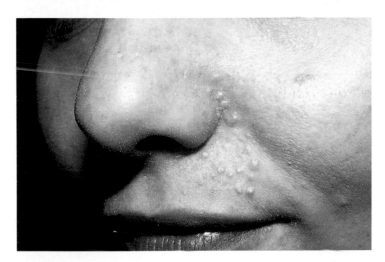

Figure 6.18

Trichoepitheliomata. Symmetrical flesh coloured papules are found in the perinasal area.

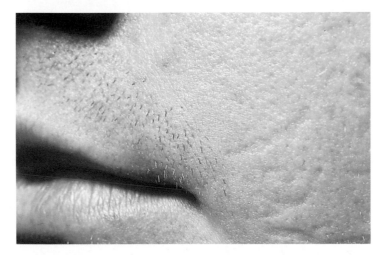

Figure 6.19

Patient with ice-pick like scars associated with atrophy. These are unrelated to acne and are called atrophia maculosa varioliformis, ulerythema ophryogenes and porphyria cutanea tarda. Other conditions implicated in scarring that are unrelated to acne include hydroavacciniformis, ulerythma ophryogenes and porphyria cutanea tarda.

7 Other acne subtypes and acne-like disorders

Introduction

Several conditions are variants of acne or are acne-related and these are discussed in this chapter. These uncommon variants appear in alphabetical order, which in no way reflects the frequency in which they are seen in the clinic.

Aggressive and severe acne

There are several forms of severe, aggressive acne.

Acne conglobata

Acne conglobata is a chronic, severe form of acne that is characterized by polyporous blackheads, burrowing abscesses and irregular scarring. Lesions may be associated with sinus tracts which often have multiple orifices, nodules and granulomatous inflammation (Figure 7.1). Males are more affected than females, and the onset is usually between the ages of 18 and 30 years. Acne conglobata frequently starts de novo but may possibly develop from existing active papular or pustular acne. The precise cause of acne conglobata is unknown but, in contrast to acne fulminans (see later), other than slight to moderate elevations of the white blood count, it is not accompanied by systemic signs or symptoms.

Polyporous blackheads are a conspicuous feature of acne conglobata. Classically appearing in pairs or groups on the neck or trunk (see Figure 7.1b), they may extend to involve the upper arms or buttocks. Inflammatory nodules form, usually in relation to the multiple comedones. The nodules gradually increase in size and break down to discharge pus. When the nodules break down, crusts may cover an indolent deep ulcer which tends to extend centrifugally with centred healing. Acne conglobata is extremely persistent and slow healing is a marked feature. Disfiguring scars, which are usually atrophic but occasionally keloidal, may accompany the progressive extension of the lesions and many cases remain active for 25 years or more.

Acne conglobata may be associated with secondary obstruction and inflammation of the apocrine units of the axilla, breast and perineum producing hidradenitis suppurativa

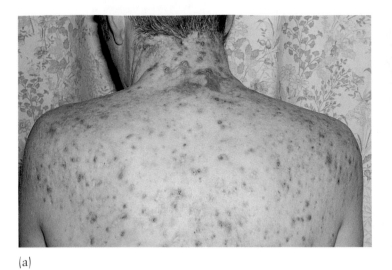

(a)

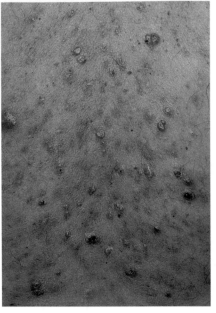

(b)

Figure 7.1

Patient with very troublesome acne conglobata. (a) Many nodules and granulomatous infiltration are present. (b) Close-up view of the polyporous blackheads

(acne inversa). Hidradenitis suppurativa is, however, more frequently associated with mild acne in typical areas. Other evidence of poral closure may be present with the patient having a pilonidal sinus and/or suppurative perifolliculis of the scalp. Treatment is notoriously difficult. Most patients are prescribed virtually every acne therapy to little avail; occasionally, however, some notable successes are achieved. Persistence is the key for both the patient and physician. Dermatosurgery with excisions of sinuses in the axillae, groin and buttocks, Z-plasty and mesh grafts or flaps are the therapy of choice in this subtype. Reduction in weight and the stopping of smoking is important.

Acne fulminans

This is an acne acute febrile reaction that is associated with severe acne, affecting males much more frequently than females. The main distinguishing features are:

- Sudden onset
- Severe and, at times, ulcerating acne (Figure 7.2)
- Usual truncal involvement (Figure 7.3)
- Systemic toxic effects as demonstrated by fever and polyarthralgia
- Failure to respond to antibacterial therapy
- Favourable response to oral steroid therapy and, after 4–6 weeks, the addition of oral isotretinoin.

The inflamed lesions often ulcerate and healing lesions are characterized by the presence of considerable granulation tissue.

The inflammatory arthralgia may affect one or several joints, especially the hips, knees and thighs, requiring the patient to be admitted to a dermatological inpatient ward. Multifocal osteolytic cysts may present as tender bones and may be detected as 'hot

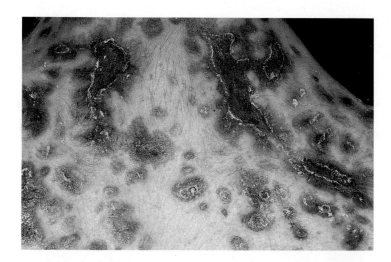

Figure 7.2

Patient with typical acne fulminans with sudden-onset ulcerating acne.

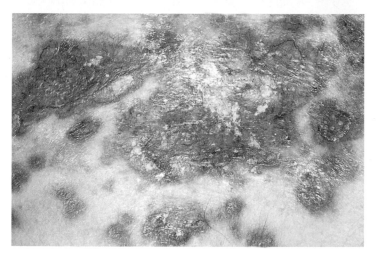

Figure 7.3

Truncal lesions in acne fulminans.

spots' using scintillography. Patients may also have erythema nodosum (Figure 7.4); in a few patients, the erythema nodosum lesions develop during isotretinoin therapy.

An elevated white blood count, with an increased percentage of polymorphonuclear leucocytes, is characteristic of this acute disorder. The haematological reaction may be very pronounced: leukaemic-type appearances have been observed. Blood cultures are almost always sterile.

The skin reactivity in acne fulminans has been monitored infrequently. One patient

with acne fulminans and erythema nodosum showed a severe necrotic reaction to an intra-dermal *P. acnes* antigen injection at 36 hours, which suggests that acne fulminans is an Arthus reaction to *P. acnes*. This was supported by intra-dermal (i.d.) testing a large series of patients from Finland. The need for oral steroids would support this view.

Genetic factors may be relevant in some instances. Four sets of identical twins have been reported to develop an identical pattern of acne fulminans, either at the same time or within 1 month of each other.

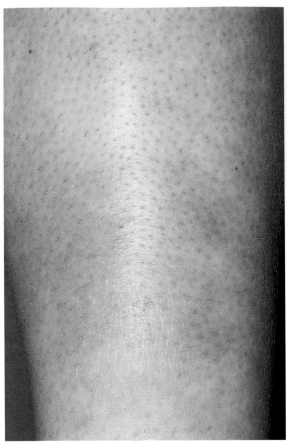

Figure 7.4

Erythema nodosum in a patient with acne
fulminans.

Gram-negative folliculitis

Gram-negative folliculitis (GNF) is an infection with gram-negative organisms that may
occur as a complication, usually during long-
term treatment of patients for acne vulgaris.
Acne patients on long-term oral antibiotic
treatment who have a sudden flare of pustular or nodular lesions, or who are considered
to be resistant to treatment, should be
sampled for GNF. This condition is an
uncommon reason for 'clinically resistant'
acne.

Although two clinical varieties of gram-
negative folliculitis are recognized, there is
much overlap. Approximately 80% of patients
with Gram-negative folliculitis have superficial pustules without comedones, which
extend from the infranasal area to the chin
and cheeks (Figure 7.5), although the lesions
can be much more widespread (Figure 7.6).
Only occasionally is the trunk involved and
very occasionally the scalp is affected (Figure
7.7). Pustular lesions are not commonly found
in ordinary acne but the occurrence of many
pustules at this site is often a useful sign that
the patient has Gram-negative folliculitis.
Enterobacteriaceae, *Klebsiella*, *Escherichia* or
Serratia genera, that is those collectively
designated as lactose-fermenting Gram-
negative rods (LFGNR), are recovered on
culture of the pustules and anterior nares.
Deep nodular lesions are seen in the remaining 20% of patients, and culture of the lesions
and anterior nares often yields *Proteus* organisms. It has also been shown that patients
with GNF may have similar organisms in
their seminal fluid. The relevance of this is
uncertain.

Overgrowth of Gram-negative enterobacte-
ria occurs only when the coagulase-negative
Gram-positive cocci and aerobic diphtheroid
are either greatly reduced in number or eradi-
cated. Usually the disease occurs with oral
antibiotic acne therapy, but very occasionally it is reported during topical antibiotic
acne therapy.

Pyoderma faciale (rosacea fulminans)

This is a rare disease that typically affects
female patients only, mainly in the 20–40
year age group. Patients present with a
sudden onset of inflammatory lesions,
usually papules and pustules (Figure 7.8).

Deep nodular lesions may also occur and
these may be interconnecting sinus tracts.

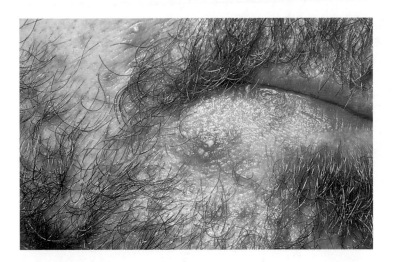

Figure 7.5

Sudden pustule development in gram-negative folliculitis.

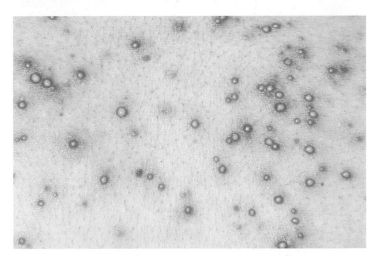

Figure 7.6

Gram-negative folliculitis: very many pustules are seen particularly on the trunk.

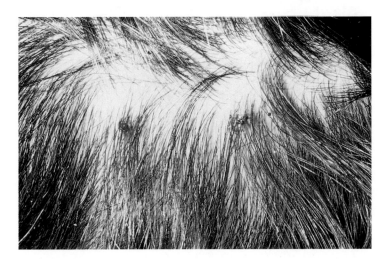

Figure 7.7

Scalp involvement with pustular lesions in Gram-negative folliculitis.

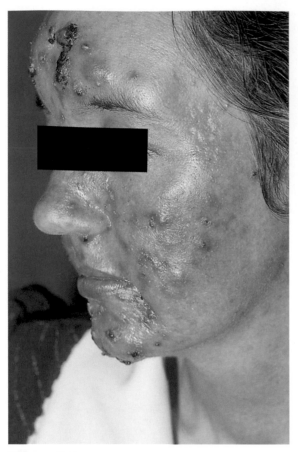

Figure 7.8

Patient with sudden onset of inflammatory facial disease called either pyoderma faciale or rosacea fulminans.

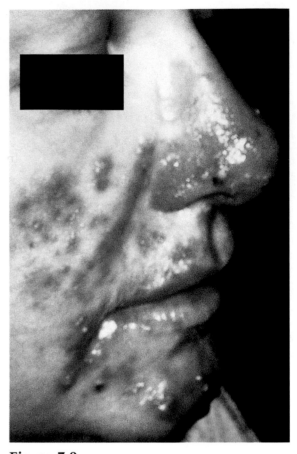

Figure 7.9

Cyanotic erythema of the face, especially centrally, in pyoderma faciale.

Typically there is a conspicuous lack of comedones and the affected area is sharply demarcated from normal skin. There is a tendency for the lesions to be localized in the central part of the face and a reddish to cyanotic erythema of the face is present (Figure 7.9)

The paranasal, malar regions and chin are almost always involved. The forehead is also frequently involved. The lateral facial areas and nasal area are usually not involved so often. Similarly, fewer patients have involve-

ment of the neck, back, chest or shoulders. A localized form of pyoderma faciale (RF), seen infrequently, involves only an isolated area such as the chin or cheek. It is probably not a separate entity but can be explained on the basis that it represents early disease.

The results of one study showed that, in most patients with rosacea fulminans (pyoderma faciale), the onset and spread of the process was rapid, occurring in less than 1 month in 75% of patients and within 1–3 months in 17%. In 8% of patients, lesions developed over a 3–6 month period. Pyoderma faciale was renamed rosacea fulminans (RF) by Kligman and Plewig because it appears to have similarities that are more common to rosacea than acne. A previous history of acne was elicited in less than 50% of patients. Controversy remains as to whether all patients with RF are patients with very severe rosacea but some patients have some features of acne. In contrast to acne fulminans, constitutional symptoms are uncommon, although, occasionally, fatigue and loss of weight are noted. Elevated leucocyte counts and sedimentation rates have been observed, not surprisingly, in some of these patients. The prominence of the lesions of pyoderma faciale can make the disease an emotionally, socially and physically devastating condition. A total of 28% of patients recalled a traumatic emotional experience before the onset of lesions.

Acne excoriée and dysmorphophobia

Acne excoriée is also called 'acne excoriée des jeunes filles'. It is predominantly a disease of young, adult women and almost always involves the face (Figure 7.10).

Patients typically 'attack' the smallest of papules.

Clinical presentation is characterized by excoriated areas of inflammation with superficial crusting.

The dividing line between acne excoriée and true neurotic excoriations (dermatitis artefacta) is tenuous, especially if the latter are confined to the face. Virtually all patients with acne excoriée have a psychiatric disorder, particularly an obsessional trait, or depression.

Psychiatric investigations have shown that in many patients the excoriations are used as

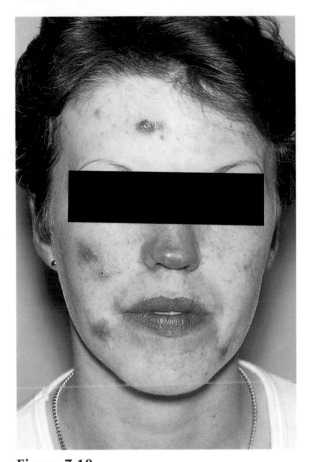

Figure 7.10

Female patient with very few acne spots, all of which have been scratched severely. This is typical of acne excoriée.

a protective device to conceal an emotional failure.

At the extreme end of the scale, patients with very mild acne, no more than one or two lesions, may present with a history of severe emotional distress. In cases such as this, their symptoms are totally out of proportion to the presenting signs (Figure 7.11). In some patients post-inflammatory pigmentation can be very striking. History taking is a very long process, since these patients have a grossly disturbed body image (dysmorphophobia) (Figure 7.12).

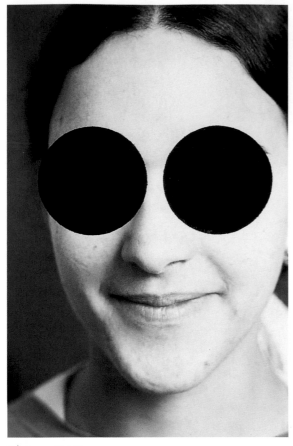

Figure 7.11

Patient with dysmorphophobia. Although only one or two lesions were present, the clinical interview took 45 minutes.

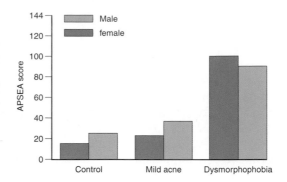

Figure 7.12

Psychological and social effects of patients with dysmorphophobia compared to patients with mild acne and a control group.

Table 7.1   Agents implicated in drug-induced acne.

Definite	*Questionable*
Androgenic hormones	Chloral hydrate
Anabolic steroids	Cyclosporin A
Oral corticosteroids	Disulfiram
Topical corticosteroids	Halothane
Lithium	Maprotiline
Halogens	Phenobarbitone
Radiation therapy	PUVA therapy
	Quinine
	Tetraethinylthiuram
	Thiouracil
	Thiourea
	Troxidone
	Vitamin B$_{12}$

Drug-induced acne

Acne can be precipitated or aggravated by certain drugs (Table 7.1).

Since the human sebaceous glands are predominantly under androgenic control, it is not surprising that testosterone can induce or aggravate acne. As would be expected, gonadotrophins, which may be prescribed for certain pituitary disorders, can aggravate acne indirectly by directly stimulating the production of testosterone.

Anabolic steroids are masculinizing and so can aggravate acne in both sexes. The most typical clinical picture of anabolic steroid acne is very severe truncal acne (Figure 7.13). This is also a problem, for example, in treating female patients with familial angiooedema with anabolic steroids. Power

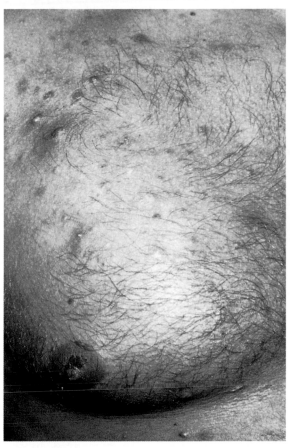

Figure 7.13

This patient was taking illicit anabolic steroids and developed very severe truncal acne.

athletes may self-administer large doses of androgenic anabolic hormones. These hormonal agents increase sebum output and so may precipitate acne. Owing to the increasing non-physician-directed usage of such anabolic steroids, these are now probably one of the commonest causes of drug-induced acne.

Oral, topical, rectal and inhaled corticosteroids and adrenocorticotrophic hormone (ACTH) can also produce iatrogenic acne. The lesions produced by corticosteroids tend to be much more monomorphic than that seen in ordinary acne. Comedones may be present (Figure 7.14) but the most common lesions are superficial papules and pustules. Nodules, cysts and scars are rare unless the patient has an underlying predisposition to acne. Flat, follicular hyperkeratotic lesions may also be seen. Steroid acne, which is dose-dependent, rarely occurs before puberty.

Halogen-induced folliculitis is now rare. The eruption often involves the face, upper trunk and the arms; comedones are rare but inflammatory lesions, especially pustules, are common and evolve rapidly. Iodides and bromides have been the main cause of halogen-induced folliculitis. Chlorine has not been found to be a cause of acneiform eruptions.

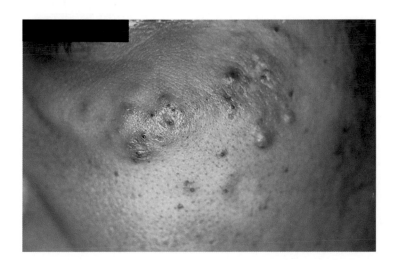

Figure 7.14

Iatrogenic acne produced by topical corticosteroid. This may be associated with inflammatory lesions and comedones, as seen here.

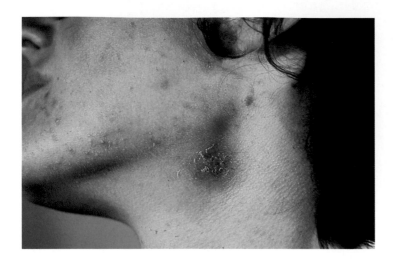

Figure 7.15

Local trauma in an acne-prone patient, particularly seen in violin and viola players (known as Fiddler's neck).

Frictional acne

Frictional acne can occur from multiple sources, depending upon the site of friction. For instance it can be seen under the headbands beneath the fur hats worn by people in cold climates, under the chin-straps worn by football players and occasionally under tight bra straps. Among musicians, fiddler's neck is reasonably well-known (Figure 7.15). This form of frictional acne also affects violin and viola players. It consists of a localized area of lichenification, just below the angle of the jaw on the neck. Papules, or pustules, are frequently present within the plaques, but nodules, cysts and scarring do not usually occur.

The mechanism of frictional acne is uncertain; it may represent a hypercornification response to local trauma or the effects of localized hydration on the pilosebaceous corneocytes.

Infantile acne

There are fundamentally two stages at which neonates and infants may present with acne or acne-like rashes – either in the first month or from the second/third month onwards. In the first month of life it is common for infants to develop monomorphic papular – pustular lesions, particularly on the cheeks. Such lesions resolve within 2–3 weeks and are of little or no concern. Although they are common, rarely does the paediatrician ask the dermatologist to see such lesions since they are recognized by the paediatrician and the primary care physician. The lesions probably result from occlusion not of the sebaceous gland duct but of the immature sweat gland duct, resulting in retention of sweat; this in turn produces a low-grade inflammation. After 2–4 weeks, however, the sweat glands begin to function normally and these benign, non-scarring lesions disappear.

Infantile or juvenile acne typically presents between the age of 3 and 18 months.

Males are affected far more than females in a ratio of 4:1. Lesions typically occur on the face and in about 1 in 20 patients on the trunk; they are clinically identical to those seen in adult acne, comprising whiteheads, blackheads, papules and pustules (Figure 7.16). Nodules and deep pustules are, however, uncommon (Figure 7.17)

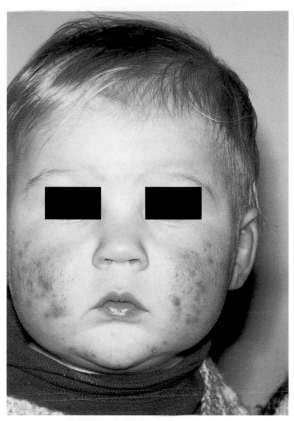

Figure 7.16

Infantile acne. Typical appearance with the presence of whiteheads, blackheads, papules and pustules.

Severe disease (Figure 7.18) will lead to scarring both of the hypertrophic, keloidal and atrophic macular variety.

The family history may reveal acne in the mother or father. How many youngsters with infantile acne go on to develop acne later on in life is not, however, really known.

Patients with infantile and juvenile acne are otherwise fit and healthy; indeed, unless there are any obvious clinical problems, there is no justification whatsoever in carrying out any blood investigations. If, however, acne persists beyond the age of 2½ years or before the age of 7 years, then one should give serious consideration to the possibility that the individual is suffering from a significant endocrinopathy, such as a hyperplasia or tumour of the gonads or adrenals.

Treatment of infantile acne is, in principle, no different from the treatment of a patient with adolescent acne. Patients with mild acne should be given topical therapy.

Topical retinoids should be used if the acne is predominantly comedonal, and benzoyl peroxide, azelaic acid or topical antibiotics if the acne is inflammatory. If the acne is of mixed appearance therapy comprises a retinoid in the morning and antimicrobial therapy in the evening

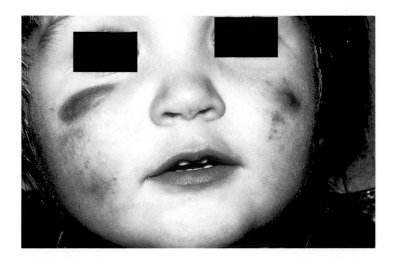

Figure 7.17

Patient with infantile acne and deeper inflammatory nodules.

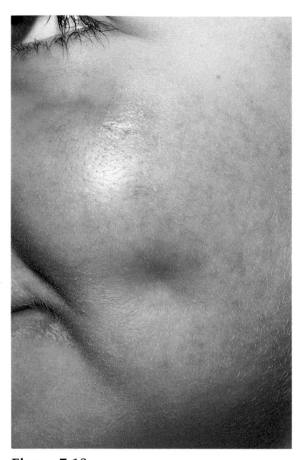

Figure 7.18

A depressed atrophic scar in an infant who had had infantile acne.

If either a patient's acne is not responding well by 3 months of such therapy or if the acne is getting worse or if the patient presents initially with moderate or severe acne, it is prudent to prescribe oral therapy in conjunction with appropriate topical therapy. Such patients should not be given oral tetracycline, doxycycline or minocycline as this will produce discolouration of the teeth. Indeed such drugs should not be given to a child below the age of 10 years. The choice is therefore usually a paediatric suspension erythromycin (125 mg bd) for a few months. If appropriate progress is not achieved it is quite likely that the child will have developed resistance of his or her *P. acnes* to the relevant antibiotic and an alternative choice will be trimethoprim (100 mg bd) in conjunction with appropriate topical therapy. Patients with mild disease will usually require therapy for 12–18 months but those with more severe disease may require oral therapy in excess of 2 years.

In exceptional cases, oral isotretinoin has been prescribed and there are now probably at least 20 patients that the authors know of who have received oral isotretinoin in a dose of 0.5 mg/kg bodyweight. Some physicians measure liver function, liver enzymes and fasting lipids prior to prescribing a 4-month course of oral isotretinoin but frequently this is not performed because of the discomfort to the child and parents. Obviously the side-effects of oral isotretinoin are similar to those that occur in adults and these also need to be shared with the family so appropriate measures can be taken to prevent or treat the relevant side-effects./

Naevoid acne

There are both structural as well as functional localized naevoid conditions involving the sebaceous elements of the follicle.

Naevus comedonicus

Naevus comedonicus is a structural alternation of the follicle that has a variety of clinical features.

Numerous investigators, depending upon whether they have emphasized the clinical or microscopic features, or both, have coined various descriptive names for this naevoid condition. Clinical naevus comedonicus is divisible into two types: in one, comedones alone are present (Figure 7.19); in the second type, inflammatory papules are also present.

The lesions are usually localized, unilateral and linear, and may be found on the scalp, face, neck, trunk and arms, and occasionally on other sites, such as the penis. Although usually present at birth, the lesions can develop much later in life. Naevus comedonicus can be a significant cosmetic problem. Chronic inflammatory lesions arise only rarely but may produce residual scarring.

In several reports, naevus comedonicus has been associated with other lesions, for example, cataract, linear basal cell naevus and epidermolytic hyperkeratosis.

Functional naevi of the sebaceous gland

This group of lesions is very uncommon. Lesions are associated with increased (or decreased) functional and structural abnormalities, predominantly involving the sebaceous glands.

Unilateral acne

This is self-explanatory; the acne being almost exclusively unilateral.

Naevoid acne

Such patients have an area of acne that is localized to one site (Figure 7.20). The area involved has an increased sebum excretion rate and evidence of increased comedogenesis on the affected site.

Non-acne naevus

Areas totally free of acne may occur with larger areas of otherwise moderate or severe

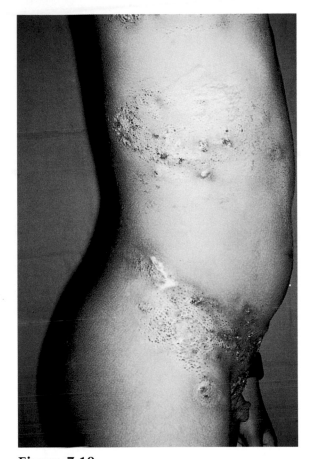

Figure 7.19

Patient with naevus comedonicus. (Courtesy of Dr D Paige.)

acne. Biopsy of the 'normal' areas shows small sebaceous follicles. These areas also have reduced sebum excretion.

Familial naevoid sebaceous gland hyperplasia

Usually, the face shows a prominent sebaceous gland hyperplasia with widened follicular openings without comedones and inflammation. The perioral and periorbital areas are not affected. An autosomal dominant trait is suspected.

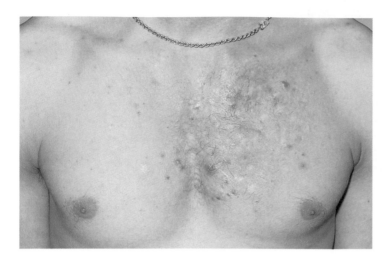

Figure 7.20

Localized acne. Acne rarely occurs in a localized faction, but it is found here as confined to one side of the body only.

Occupational acne

Chloracne

Chloracne is an acneiform eruption resulting from halogenated aromatic compounds with a specific molecular shape. It is a syndrome characterized by the presence of comedones, especially on the face (Figure 7.21) of various sizes. Inflammation is usually mild when considering the extent of the comedonal components. Common chlorocnegens are:

- Chloronapththalenes (CNs)
- Polychlorinated biphenyls (PCBs)
- Polychlorinated dibenzofurans (PCDFs), especially tri-, tetra-, penta- and hexachlorodibenzofuran
- Contaminants of chlorophenols:
  - 2,3,7,8-Tetrachlorodibenzo-p-dioxin (TCDD)
  - Hexachlorodibenzo-p-dioxin
  - Tetrachlorodibenzofuran
- Chlorobenzenes
  - Crude trichlorobenzene
  - Crude benzene hexachloride
  - 3,4,3′,4′ Tetrachlorozoxybenzene

Chloracne has also been caused, uncommonly, by brominated biphenyls. The clinical features of chloracne are listed in Table 7.2.

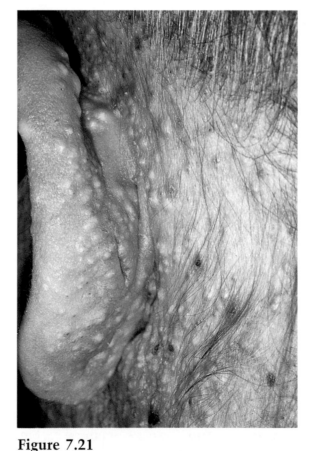

Figure 7.21

Patient with multiple comedones, typical of chloracne.

Table 7.2 Clinical features of chloracne.

Mucocutaneous	*Systemic*
Chloracne and cysts	Hepatic dysfunction
Melanin pigmentation	Raised triglycerides
Hypertrichosis	Hepatic porphyria
Phrynoderma	Bronchitis
Erythema	Nervous system involvement
Palmar and plantar hyperhidrosis	Long-term predisposition to cancer
Conjunctivitis: blepharitis	

Treatment is difficult; topical retinoids or gentle cautery under local anaesthetic ENLA® may help. Oral and topical antibiotics do, to some extent, control the inflammatory acne. However, oral isotretinoin is of no benefit.

Oil acne

A variety of oil products may cause acneiform eruptions. In the past, industrial contact with cutting oils was quite common but, as industrial hygiene has improved and good manufacturing conditions have been instituted, oil folliculitis is seen less frequently. Oil folliculitis is more likely to appear on covered areas such as the thighs where there is likely to have been prolonged contact with oil saturated clothing. The involved individuals have follicular papules and pustules (Figure 7.22). In severe cases, furuncle-like lesions are present and these heal with scars. The mechanism of the disease is unknown but it is believed to be related to the mechanical obstruction and penetration of oils into the follicle.

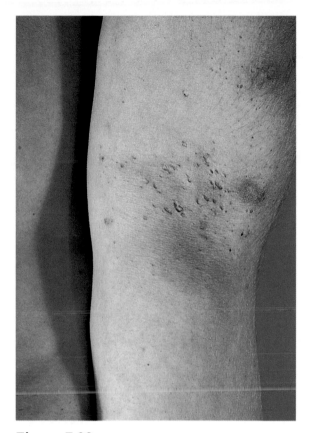

Figure 7.22

Oil acne induced by external oil products in an atypical area, here cubital area of the left arm.

Pomade and cosmetic acne

Pomade acne (Figure 7.23) is more commonly encountered in the USA than in Europe. Pomade acne is an acneiform eruption that occurs on the forehead and temple. It consists mainly of uniform closed comedones, with occasional papules and pustules. This eruption typically occurs in Afro-Caribbeans who apply pomades to straighten their hair. It probably represents a special type of oil acne. A reduction in the use of pomades is associated with a gradual reduction in the pomade acne.

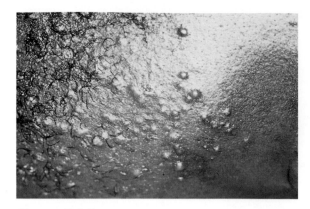

Figure 7.23

Afro-Caribbean patient with typical pomade acne. Multiple similar looking whiteheads are present.

As many as one-third of American females in the age range 20–50, years especially between the ages of 20–30 years, have been reported as having a very mild form of papular acne. It has been suggested that cosmetics are the cause of this type of acne. The lesions are situated predominantly on the cheeks and around the mouths. Most of the lesions are papular. Comedones may be present but pustules are rare. Premenstrual exacerbations and seborrhoea are not features of this form of acne.

Animal experiments, although overpredictive compared with the human situation, have shown that certain cosmetics and their components are comedogenic.

Actinic (senile) comedones

It is common to find large comedones in the loose tissues around the orbit and malar regions of elderly individuals (Figure 7.24). They occur particularly in those who have been exposed to excessive amounts of ultra-violet radiation and nicotine, in whom these comedones may also be seen on the neck. Solar damage to the supporting collagen tissue is probably an essential part in their development. As a result of the damaged collagen tissue, the pilosebaceous duct is more easily distended by impacted corneocytes.

Syndromes associated with acne

Such associations are rare and include Apert's syndrome (acrophalangosyndactyly), which is the association of short stature, short and fused digits (Figure 7.25a) and, in most patients, a flattened face. Clinical findings in nine patients with Apert's syndrome revealed seven postpubertal patients to have moderate to severe acne vulgaris on the face, chest, back and also, in an unusual manner, the forearms (Figure 7.25b). The bony features of this syndrome result from premature epiphyseal closure; this phenomenon and acne are both androgen-mediated. It is suggested that the syndrome represents an end-organ hyper-response to androgens.

Acne in these patients is usually relatively therapy resistant and often requires oral isotretinoin.

Hidradenitis suppurativa-like acne (acne inversa)

Hidradenitis suppurativa, which is sometimes associated with acne, is a chronic, cicatrizing, suppurative disorder of the regions bearing apocrine glands.

The association with acne vulgaris, which is established as a condition dependent on androgens, the failure of hidradenitis suppurativa to develop before puberty, and the general decline in disease activity at the

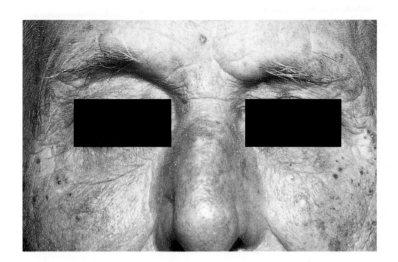

Figure 7.24

An elderly patient who has got much loss of collagen and dystended ducts, resulting in solar comedones.

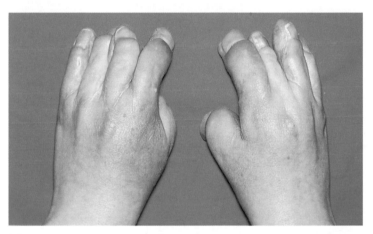

(a)

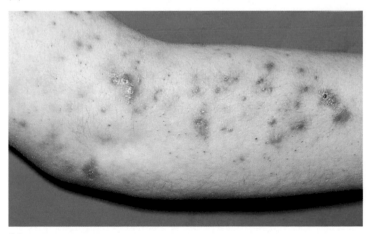

(b)

Figure 7.25

(a) Patient with fused digits typical of Apert's syndrome. (b) Unusual distribution of acne on the forearms in Apert's syndrome.

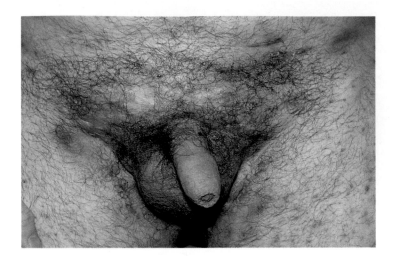

Figure 7.26

Troublesome hidradenitis is present in the genitocrural area.

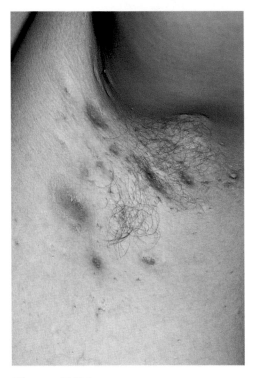

Figure 7.27

Hidradenitis suppurativa. Significant inflammatory nodular scarring disease is present.

menopause all suggest a condition dependent on hormones. In over 60% of cases of hidradenitis suppurativa there is often a family history of hidradenitis. It should not be misdiagnosed with a true primary infection with staphylococci of the sweat glands originating from the epidermal acrosyringium (porus) later penetrating the depth of the sweat gland. Compared with acne it is a much less-investigated disease.

The disease affects apocrine sites, namely the axilla, anogenital area and breasts (Figure 7.26); some sites may be involved more than others.

Although many of the lesions are papules and pustules, the major lesions are inflammatory nodules (Figure 7.27) which may become quite large.

The presence of sinus tracts is common, with much discharge of foul-smelling pus. Scarring is common (Figure 7.28).

In one series, 47.5% of patients had significant acne and 17% were hirsute. Blackheads were found in apocrine sites in 88% but also in retroauricular sites in 43%: these were considered to be an important physical sign for early diagnosis. Pilonidal sinuses were evident in 19%.

Patients with hidradenitis suppurativa are likely to be seen not only by dermatologists

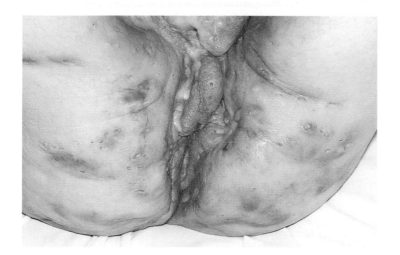

Figure 7.28

Scarring in patient with hidradenitis suppurativa.

but also by general and plastic surgeons, and gynaecologists. The disease is often at an advanced stage before it is diagnosed, by which time undermining abscesses and sinus tracts have become established. The magnitude of the social, economic and medical problems confronting these patients is not generally recognized. Although the disease can become spontaneously quiescent at an early state, it more commonly continues relentlessly for years.

Successful treatment is unusual. Patients try repeat and prolonged courses of antibiotics, Dianette®, oral isotretinoin and oral and topical steroids, often with little benefit. Many patients are treated with local excision of lesions; wider excision (Figures 7.29–7.32) or CO_2 laser abrasion of the apocrine sites in the axillae and groin is usually preferred to having repeated local excision.

Tropical acne

During World War II and the Korean and Vietnam conflicts, many of the allied troops serving in South East Asia either had an exacerbation of the pre-existing acne, or

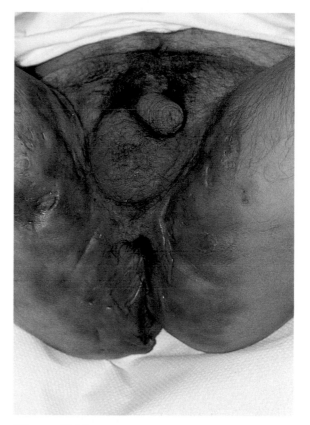

Figure 7.29

Severe acne inversa (hidradenitis suppurativa) with significant inflammatory nodular lesions and draining sinuses.

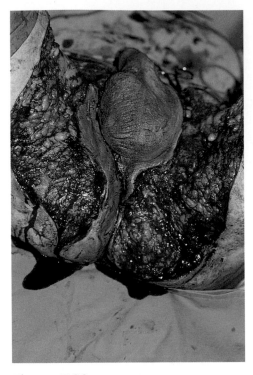

Figure 7.30

The same patient after dermatosurgery with total eradication of the fistulae, sinuses and chronic inflammatory pachydermic tissue.

developed acne de novo. The severity of the disease was such that it was a common cause of non-traumatic medical evacuation. Tropical acne is often a very inflammatory type of acne, and is most prevalent on the trunk, extending down onto the arms. Changes in ductal corneocyte hydration are implicated; these, in turn, accentuate blockage of the pilosebaceous duct, increasing sebum outflow resistance and thereby potentiating acne.

A similar situation to tropical acne is seen in workers in hot, humid situations, who also tend to suffer from flares of inflammatory acne.

Tropical acne may also be aetiologically related to acne aestivale (Majorca acne) seen in patients who have recently returned from a holiday in a sunny and humid environment. Additional external comedogenic factors such as sunscreen oils may also be important. The lesions are usually

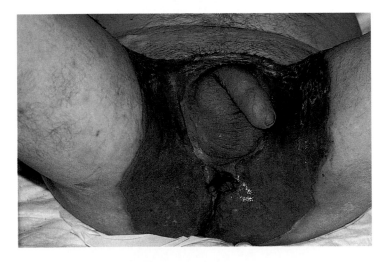

Figure 7.31

The same patient during granulation of tissue and first transplantation of mesh-grafts.

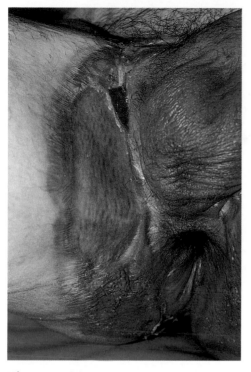

Figure 7.32

The same patient after additional one month demonstrating a good wound healing without any acne inversa like lesions.

monomorphic, consisting of small inflamed lesions intermixed with non-inflamed lesions. The level of inflammation is less than that seen in tropical acne, probably owing to a shorter duration of exposure (Figure 7.33).

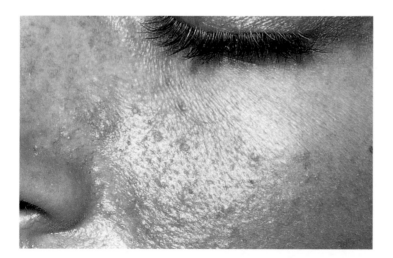

Figure 7.33

Patient with typical 'Majorca acne'. Within 2 weeks of a sunny humid holiday and the use of many particularly oily sunscreens, acute monomorphic acne lesions developed.

Part III: Types of therapy and management approaches

8 Topical therapy

Introduction

The importance to which topical therapy is included in the management of acne depends upon the severity of the disease. Topical therapy is usually all that is needed for most cases of mild to mild-moderate acne (Figures 8.1 and 8.2) in the management of more severe disease. Topical acne therapy is then used in combination with oral therapy (except isotretinoin) in moderate to severe cases with more inflammation and a tendency to scar and, finally, is also used as maintenance therapy once the disease is brought under good control. As with systemic therapy, the choice of agents used for topical therapy is dependent upon the clinical presentation and the general principles of therapy. These general principles of treatment are to:

- Decrease sebaceous gland secretion
- Correct the altered patterns of ductal hypercornification
- Decrease the population of *P. acnes* and the generation of extracellular inflammatory products by *P. acnes*
- Produce an anti-inflammatory effect

No topical therapy currently available has been found to decrease the seborrhoea. Before choosing the topical therapy, a good examination of the skin is critical. It is impossible to choose intelligently the appropriate topical therapeutic agent without determining whether a patient has non-inflammatory acne, inflammatory acne, or a mixture of non-inflammatory and inflammatory lesions. One of the major advances in topical therapy has been the tailoring of therapy to the status of the disease.

An overview of the mechanism of action of the most commonly prescribed topical agents is given in Table 8.1.

Table 8.1 The therapeutic action of topical agents.

	Anti-comedogenic	Anti-microbial	Anti-inflammatory
Salicylic acid	±	–	±
Benzoyl peroxide	±	++	±
Antibiotics	+	++	+
Azelaic acid	+	+	+
Tretinoin	++	±	–
Isotretinoin	++	±	±
Tazarotene	++	±	–
Adapalene	++	±	+
Retinaldehyde	+	±	±

–, No effect; ±, possible effect; +, some effect; ++, moderate effect.

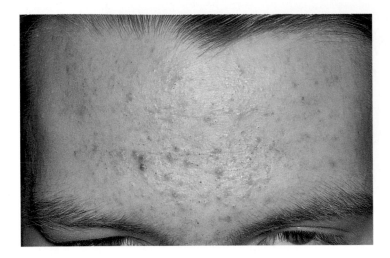

Figure 8.1

Mild acne needing topical therapy alone.

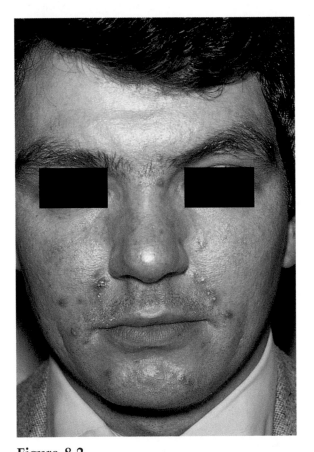

Figure 8.2

Mild–moderate acne needing topical therapy alone.

Most topical agents can be classified according to whether they act upon the process of ductal hypercornification or through an antibacterial action. In general, for non-inflammatory (comedonal) acne the use of agents with anticomedogenic properties is appropriate, whereas in inflammatory acne agents that are antibacterial are indicated. This dictum cannot be followed absolutely, however. Firstly, most cases of acne are not monomorphic except in early acne, which tends to be primarily comedonal, most cases having a mixed-lesion pattern. Furthermore, many clinical studies have shown that there is a reduction in comedones in patients treated with agents such as benzoyl peroxide antibiotics and, similarly, there are reductions in inflammatory lesions in patients treated with the various topical retinoids and similar drugs.

Choice of topical therapy

Choice of topical therapy depends upon acne severity and skin type. Severity is not just related to the number of lesions, however, it depends on other factors such as:

Table 8.2 Classification of acne severity according to number and types of lesions.

Severity	Comedones	Papules/pustules	Nodules, 'cysts', sinus tracts	Inflammation	Scarring
Mild	<10	<10	–	–	–
Moderate	<20	>10–50	–	+	±
Severe	>20–50	>50–100	≤5	++	++
Very severe	>50 and/or directly fused comedones	>100	>5	+++	+++

–, none; ±, variable; +, mild-moderate; ++, considerable; +++, extensive

- Distribution – the acne may be localized or generalized
- Degree of inflammation (Figures 8.3 and 8.4)
- Duration of disease
- Previous response to therapy
- Psychosocial effects of the disease.

In the clinic, overall physical severity can be assessed by reference to standard photographs. These are shown in greater detail in Chapter 5.

An easy to follow classification of acne grading based on the number and types of lesions is shown in Table 8.2.

General advice

Before starting any therapy in acne, each patient should be told to apply topical therapy not only to the lesion itself, but also

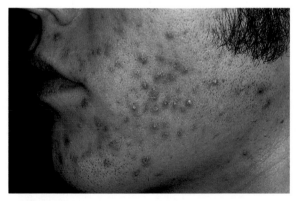

Figure 8.3

Papular–pustular acne of moderate type. Inflammatory lesions predominate. Topical treatment preferentially with benzoyl peroxide and/or topical antibiotics or azelaic acid is indicated. In addition, oral antibiotics are likely to be required.

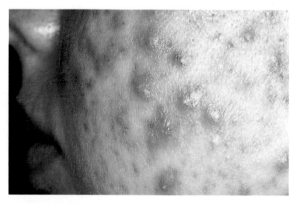

Figure 8.4

Papular–pustular acne with small indurated lesions. The start of the formation of small nodules stresses the need for combined oral treatment and topical therapy.

to all areas of skin that are predisposed to acne vulgaris. This is most important since the so-called normal follicles may, indeed, be microcomedones histologically and may be colonized with *P. acnes*.

It is essential to emphasize to the patient the need for maximum compliance, since the therapeutic success is highly dependent on a regular application of topical agents over a prolonged period of time. It may take years for the acne to resolve and so topical therapies need to be used for the whole of the acne 'life'. In mild physical disease this may be 2–4 years but, in more severe disease, for up to 12 years. If, however, the patient went on to be plagued with the disease persistently into the fourth decade then therapy for up to 30 years may be required. It is also necessary to encourage the patient to treat the trunk. Application to the back is not easy but usually some help is at hand from a mother, boyfriend or girlfriend and so on. In the beginning, topical acne therapy requires an active, intensive management, followed by a period of maintenance and prevention.

Side-effects and contra-indications of topical therapy

When choosing and prescribing a topical agent, possible side effects and contraindications must be remembered and discussed with the patient. A summary of possible side-effects is given in Table 8.3.

Side-effects

Most topical therapies produce a low-grade irritant dermatitis (Figures 8.5 and 8.6), indeed the lack of dermatitis should alert the physician to possible non-compliance. An allergic Type IV dermatitis is extremely rare. Other side-effects can occur, namely:

- A yellow skin fluorescence with topical tetracycline
- Bleaching of the clothes with benzoyl peroxide
- Very rare skin fragility with retinoids
- Topical antibiotics may induce *P. acnes* resistance.

Table 8.3 **Adverse drug reactions of topical therapeutics.**

Agent	Erythema	Scaling	Burning	Flare-up of acne	Bacterial resistance	Photo-sensitivity	Other
Retinoids							
– All-trans retinoic acid	+++	+++	++	++	–	++	Skin fragility – v. rare
– Isotretinoin	++	++	+	+	–	+	
– Adapalene	+	+	+	+	–	–	
Azelaic acid	+	+	++	–	–	–	–
Benzoyl peroxide	++	++	+	+	–		Bleaches hair and clothes; contact allergy is rare
Topical antibiotics	±	±	±	±	+++	Tetra-cyclines	Contact allergy, bacterial resistance

–, none; +, mild; ++, considerable; +++, extensive.

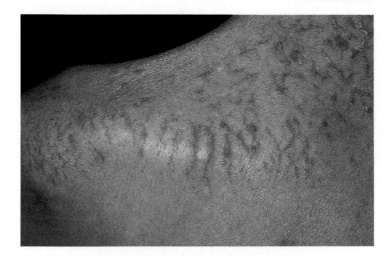

Figure 8.5

Moderate grade irritant dermatitis produced by combined treatment with all-trans-retinoic-acid and benzoylperoxide.

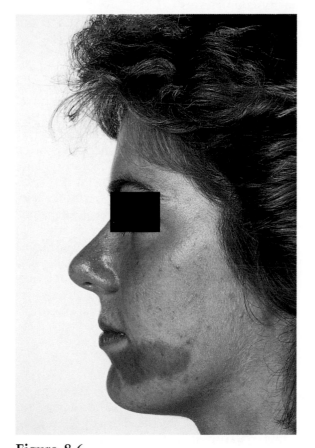

Figure 8.6

Low-grade irritant dermititis produced by benzoyl peroxide.

Contraindications of topical therapy

Any topical retinoids are currently contra-indicated during pregnancy.

Although not contraindicated, the use of azelaic acid is not recommended during pregnancy.

Topical therapies available

A brief description of the topical therapies is now presented.

Retinoids

Retinoids have been used for over 30 years, since the 1960s, when Stüttgen and Baer discovered that retinoic acid significantly affected disorders of keratinization.

Retinoids are taken up by keratinocytes and/or sebocytes, depending on the type, and are transcribed after binding to specific receptors. The activation and inhibition of certain steps of gene transcription results in changes of different pathways. These pathways include proliferation, differentiation, inflammation and sebum production.

In contrast to other retinoids, retinoids that are used topically to treat acne vulgaris finally lead to a reduced production of keratohyalin granules by follicular keratinocytes. This event may be related to a decrease in comedone formation. In addition, topical retinoids modulate in vitro macroaggregation of keratin filaments, resulting in a decrease of the coherence of keratinocytes in the comedone.

Some retinoids such as tretinoin increases the mitotic activity of the ductal keratinocytes; this leads to an increased turnover of the infundibular keratinocytes, resulting in an accelerated protrusion of the comedone. These studies were performed many years ago. This mechanism does not necessarily fit with the concept that in acne comedones there is already hyperproliferation of ductal keratinocytes. Recently research efforts focused not only on developing less irritating formulations for all-trans-retinoic-acid such as a gel microsphere formulation and a formulation in which tretinoin is incorporated into a polymer but also newly synthesized molecules with less irritating potential.

Tretinoin (all-trans-retinoic acid)

Tretinoin was the first topical retinoid used in acne and remained the gold standard for many years. It is usually available as gels or creams. More recently there has been an increase in sophistication in that several new formulations have been developed such as microsponges or propolymers.

Isotretinoin (13-cis-retinoic acid)

The effect of isotretinoin when topically applied is quite different from the effects of systemic application, since the topical use of isotretinoin does not reduce the sebum secretion rate. When topically applied, it has similar properties to tretinoin but it causes less skin irritation.

Topical isotretinoin is available as a 0.1% cream or gel, either alone or in combination with erythromycin or clindamycin.

Motretinid

Motretinid is a monoaromatic second-generation retinoid. Although less effective than tretinoin, it causes less local irritation than tretinoin. Motretinid is not available in many countries.

Adapalene

Adapalene has been on the market in several countries for up to 3 years. It is a novel retinoid, that not only reduces comedones, but produces various anti-inflammatory effects. Such clinical data has been supported by fairly respectable in vitro laboratory data. Extensive clinical studies show it to be as equally effective as all-trans retinoic acid; however, one major advantage of adapalene seems to be a considerable reduction in many of the side-effects seen with all-trans retinoic acid. This factor might make it a preferred choice in clinical practice; ultimately, the clinicians will decide its appropriate place in patient management.

Tazarotene

Tazarotene, a topical retinoid used in psoriasis and acne, is released to the market for these indications in the United States. In comparison to adapalene the treatment with tazarotene is associated with a slightly higher transient increase in peeling, erythema and dryness during the first few weeks of treatment. The efficacy of tazarotene 0.1% gel has been compared with tretinoin 0.05% gel in a multicentre double-blind randomized parallel-group trial in mild to moderate acne vulgaris for up to 12 weeks. From this data it seems that tazarotene is more efficacious than tretinoin in reducing papules and open comedones. The efficacy in reducing the number of closed comedones was similar.

Retinalaldehyde 0.1%

Recently a randomized clinical trial with retinalaldehyde 0.1% and erythromycin in mild acne vulgaris showed a significant improvement of the combination on comedones, but not with topical erythromycin alone. Some evidence suggests that retinalaldehyde has some antibacterial effects.

Retinoyl-Beta-Glucoronide (RBG)

Retinoyl-beta-glucoronide cream was recently reported to be effective in mild acne in patients of Caucasian and Indian skin type in two clinical trials. It is not yet available in most of the countries. Similar to retinalaldehyde it may become a topical retinoid for mild comedonic and less inflammatory acne.

Azelaic acid

Azelaic acid is a C9-dicarbonic acid, which is produced naturally by *M. furfur*. It is available as a 20% cream and is recommended in cases of mild and mild–moderate acne. Azelaic acid reduces the number of comedones: partly because it reduces the production of keratohylalin granules in ductal keratinocytes.

The antimicrobiotic effect of azelaic acid is based on a reduction of the colonization with *P. acnes* on the skin surface and the pilosebaceous duct. Azelaic acid produces a reduction in *P. acnes* of the order of 1 log. An anti-inflammatory effect has been suggested as a result of a decreased production of reactive oxygen specimens by polymorphonuclear leucocytes, when exposed to azelaic acid.

One advantage of azelaic acid is its relative lack of significant side-effects in particular bacterial resistance. Comparative studies show it to be equally effective as benzoyl peroxide, topical erythromycin and oral erythromycin.

Benzoyl peroxide

Benzoyl peroxide is an effective topical agent that has been used in acne vulgaris therapy for 30 years or more. It is available in different concentrations (2.5%, 4%, 5% and 10%), and different formulations such as gels, creams and lotions. It acts predominantly through its antimicrobial effects on *P. acnes*, which are reduced by about 2 log cycles. The anti-inflammatory effects of benzoyl peroxide could be the result of a reduction of oxygen radicals. It is not sebosuppressive. Benzoyl peroxide often induces an irritant dermatitis; a true allergic contact dermatitis is rare, with an incidence being less than 1:500.

Topical antibiotics

Many topical antibiotic formulations are available, either alone or in combination. Antibiotics currently and commonly used are tetracycline, erythromycin and clindamycin. A gyrase inhibitor (quinolone) is just becoming available in some countries.

The antimicrobial effect is due to a reduction in lesions of skin surface and follicular

P. acnes. A most important side-effect of topical antibiotics is the induction of bacterial resistance and cross-resistance. There has been a dramatic increase in resistance over the past 20 years. Whether this is a result of topical or oral antibiotic therapy, or both, is unknown. There is evidence that combined therapy with either zinc, benzoyl peroxide increases the bacterial effect and reduces the risk of resistance.

Other topical therapies

Salicylic acid is used in some countries in 1–3% alcoholic solutions. Besides astringent effects, keratolytic effects on the interfollicular epidermis and the acroinfundibulum may be observed. Sulphur-containing preparations are rarely used. Recently, hydrogen peroxide cream was compared with fusidic acid in impetigo. This new cream formulation stabilizes hydrogen peroxide avoiding fast degradation with the result of a prolonged antimicrobial effect. The formulation is based on crystalline lipids. It has good antibacterial effects against Gram-positive as well as Gram-negative bacteria. It may therefore be an additional topical treatment for patients with Gram-negative folliculitis.

Topical antiandrogens are unavailable because the systemic effects on the sebocytes could never be demonstrated via the topical route. An Italian study showed an efficacy of spironolactone 2% in a cream base, but could not be confirmed by the authors.

Ultraviolet radiation is used by very few dermatologists. UVA-light may be comedogenic, because squalene is oxidized to squalene peroxide, which in turn may irritate the follicular keratocytes. Conversely, UVB wavelengths probably camouflage the inflammatory aspects of acne. Very recently, it was demonstrated that ultraviolet radiation around the wavelengths of 420–460 nm activates porphyrins that are released by *P. acnes*, which then help to destroy the bacteria itself.

9 Systemic therapy

In the treatment of acne, the three major groups of oral therapy are antibiotics, hormones and retinoids. Antibiotics are usually the first line of oral therapy.

Oral therapy is indicated in subjects with moderate and severe acne (Figure 9.1). It is also prescribed for patients with mild acne who show evidence of scarring and/or are psychologically very depressed (Figure 9.2). It may also be prescribed for patients for whom employment is difficult because of their acne, even if the acne is relatively mild. Black-skinned patients tend to develop postinflammatory macules (Figure 9.3) which may last for many months; thus oral therapies are often indicated in such patients, even if the acne is otherwise mild. Oral antibiotics and hormonal anticonceptives are usually combined with topical agents.

Once initiated, oral therapy must be maintained for several months or even years. For oral antibiotics, a minimum of 6–12 months is required and this must be emphasized to the patient. Hormonal therapy is frequently prescribed for 1–6 years. Isotretinoin is usually prescribed for 4 months but occasionally a little longer. Repeat courses of all therapies can be re-prescribed if appropriate.

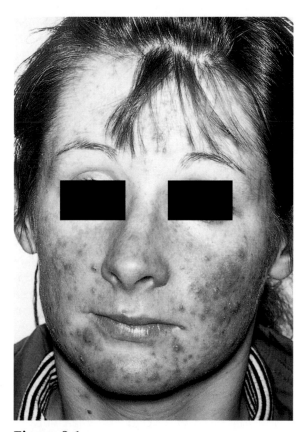

Figure 9.1

A patient with moderate acne who clearly needs oral therapy, possibly combined with topical therapy.

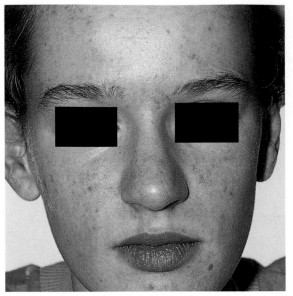

Figure 9.2

Patient with very mild acne in whom the interview was long because the patient had altered body image or dysmorphophobia. Such patients require oral therapy.

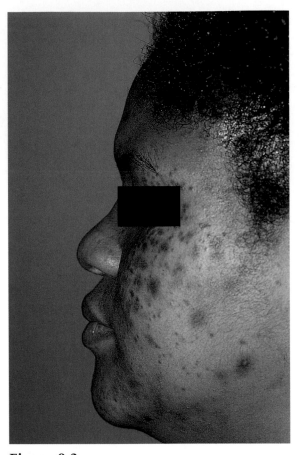

Figure 9.3

An Asiatic patient who, following mild acne, has developed very significant postinflammatory macules. These may last for several months.

Antibiotics

Somewhat disappointingly, there are only a few dose-response studies of acne treatment with antibiotics and there is a remarkable lack of evidence-based medicine. Tetracycline still remains and should remain the first choice. Minocycline is expensive but valuable in tetracycline resistant non-responsive cases. Doxycycline is a less expensive alternative but patients with tetracycline resistant *P. acnes* are likely to have *P. acnes* that is resistant to doxycycline. Erythromycin is widely used by primary care physicians but *P. acnes* that is resistant to erythromycin is an increasing problem. It is the drug of choice in a patient allergic to tetracycline, or in a female who is contemplating pregnancy, or in the treatment of a pregnant patient with severe acne who requires oral therapy. Trimethoprim is a third-line alternative. Co-trimoxazole, once used particularly in Gram-negative folliculitis, should now no longer be prescribed because it is more toxic than trimethoprim alone. Trimethoprim should also be considered for patients who do not respond to tetracycline, minocycline or erythromycin, or who are intolerant of such preparations.

Tetracycline

Tetracycline is the first choice in oral therapy and must be taken 30–60 minutes before food, preferably with water. This does not encourage compliance. If the patient is on iron or antacids, such therapies must be taken after food. Calcium, iron and antacids prescribed with tetracycline reduce absorption of the tetracycline. Dose-response studies have demonstrated that the recommended dose is 1 g/day given in two divided doses. There is probably no justification for smaller doses.

Erythromycin

Erythromycin is less affected by food but produces more gastrointestinal intolerance. It is not a preferred first-line therapy because of its *P. acnes* resistant profile.

Minocycline

Minocycline, a variant of tetracycline, is very well absorbed compared with tetracycline and can be taken with food. It may have a more rapid effect in the resolution of inflammatory acne lesions and has a greater effect in reducing surface *P. acnes* than tetracycline. Minocycline (100 mg/day) should not be the first choice for the acne patient but could be considered in a patient not responding to tetracycline. Resistance to *P. acnes* is rare. In patients not responding, the dose can be increased to 150 mg or 200 mg/day. However, it should be noted that minocycline is easier to take as it can be taken with food. Minocycline is quite expensive in some countries.

Doxycycline

A further alternative in the tetracycline group is doxycycline at a dose of 100 mg/day. Studies have shown it to be equally effective as minocycline. Doxycycline should be taken with food and a glass of water, otherwise there is a risk of oesophagitis. Patients whose *P.acnes* are resistant to tetracycline are also resistant to doxycycline, thus it is likely to be a less effective drug than it was some years ago.

Trimethoprim

Studies have shown trimethoprim (400 mg/day) to be as effective as tetracycline in the average acne patient requiring oral therapy. Doses of up to 300 mg bd can be given if needed. It is also reasonably effective in Gram-negative folliculitis but not so successful as oral isotretinoin.

Mechanism of action of antibiotics

The mechanism of action of oral antibiotics is predominantly antimicrobial. Antimicrobial drugs, which are of help clinically, significantly reduce *P. acnes*.

Doses of 1 g of tetracycline and erythromycin suppress the number of surface *P. acnes* by 1–2 log cycles. The reduction in *P. acnes* numbers is not so large as that seen with topical benzoyl peroxide and yet, in the moderately severe patient, oral antibiotics are a preferred choice, although frequently prescribed in combination with topical therapies. It is therefore quite likely that an important mechanism of oral antibiotics is achieved through non-antimicrobial anti-inflammatory effects. Several mechanisms are possible, including a reduction in inflammatory cytokines, reduction in chemotaxis to *P. acnes* by modification of complement pathways and by affecting oxygen radicals. The dose of tetracycline required to decrease *P. acnes*-stimulated chemotaxis is less than that required to suppress the number of *P. acnes*.

P. acnes *resistance*

Further evidence for the role of *P. acnes* in triggering inflammatory acne is a relationship between the development of *P. acne* resistance and the lack of clinical effect to the appropriate antibiotic, be that oral or topical in some patients.

Prior to 1980 very few *P. acnes* were resistant to commonly used antibiotics but, in the past 5 years there has been a dramatic increase in the level of resistance to *P. acnes* (Figure 9.4). In a hospital-based practice in the UK it is 67%.

Within this resistant group, the resistance varies with different antibiotics. The main antibiotics so incriminated are erythromycin and clindamycin (60%) and there has been an increase of resistance to tetracycline over the past 2 years which is now 22% (Figure 9.5). In 18% of patients there are mixed resistances. Resistance to minocycline is rare (<2%).

Common side-effects of oral antibiotic therapy

Gastrointestinal side-effects

Nausea is uncommon and vomiting is rare. Relatively mild abdominal colic with or without mild diarrhoea occurs in 6% of patients. This is usually intermittent, often requiring no treatment but, if necessary, loperamide (4 mg bd for 1–5 days), repeated when necessary usually controls the side-effects.

Severe diarrhoea resulting from pseudomembranous colitis has not been seen by the authors. It has, however, been reported with tetracycline, erythromycin and clindamycin, but it is exceedingly rare.

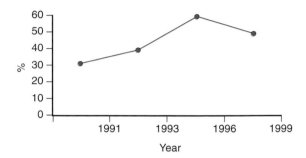

Figure 9.4

The increase in *P. acnes* resistance with time.

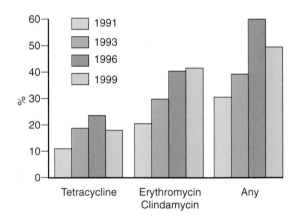

Figure 9.5

The variable resistance of *P. acnes* to a variety of antibiotics. Resistance is seen particularly with erythromycin and clindamycin. Resistance to minocycline is rare.

Vaginal candidiasis

This occurs in 2.5% of patients but is virtually limited to sexually active female patients. However, it is important to treat both partners. A stool examination of increased candida quantities in females is sometimes recommended if frequent relapses occur.

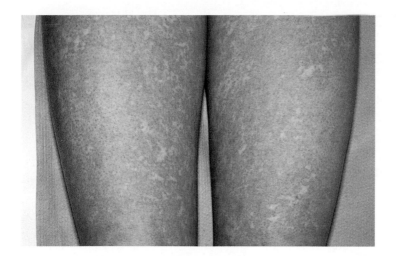

Figure 9.6

An acute drug rash caused by trimethoprim antibiotic therapy.

Drug rash

A drug rash may occur with any drug. The commonest antibiotic drug rash seen in acne is with trimethoprim (5%) therapy (Figure 9.6). Localized fixed drug rashes occur very infrequently, particularly with tetracycline.

Uncommon side-effects of antibiotic therapy

Benign intracranial hypertension

This is particularly seen with minocycline. It presents as headache, dizziness, nausea and, in extreme cases, blurred vision due to papilloedema. The patient needs to be told of these side-effects as the problem can be serious if the patient continues with the therapy. If the patient stops therapy within a few days then there are no sequelae.

Pigmentation

Minocycline produces a dose-dependent pigmentation that occurs especially in acne scars. It usually disappears within 18 months of stopping therapy. It can affect acne and other scars (Figure 9.7) and the mucosae (Figure 9.7c). Resolution of cutaneous lesions can be aided by the Q-switch ruby laser (Figure 9.8).

Phototoxicity

Doxycycline is associated with dose-dependent phototoxicity (Figure 9.9).

Autoimmune disease

Minocycline may also produce two types of autoimmune disorder. One occurs usually at 3 months and may consist of a fever, arthralgia, hepatitis and pneumonitis. The second type occurs at 10–12 months and consists of a lupus erythromatosus (LE)-like illness (including the LE rash) hepatitis and arthralgia. As with any significant side-effect therapy should be stopped.

Tetracyclines should not be given to patients with a personal or family history of LE.

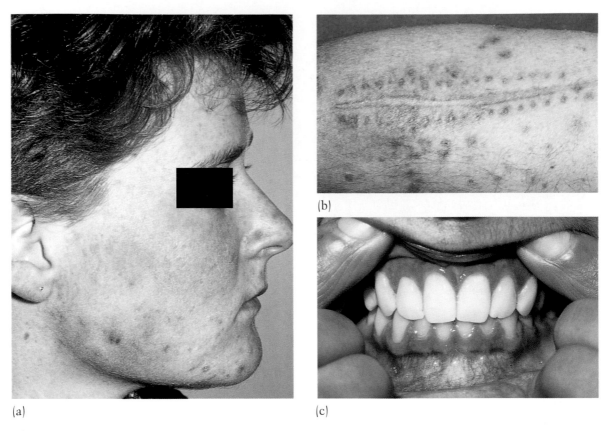

(a)

(b)

(c)

Figure 9.7

Minocycline pigmentation: (a) in acne scars; (b) in scars outside the acne sites; (c) in the mucous membranes of the mouth.

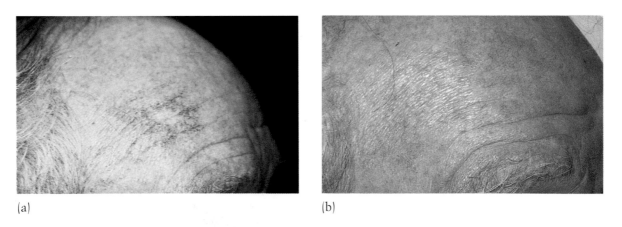

(a)

(b)

Figure 9.8

Patient with rosacea treated with minocycline; (a) who developed minocycline pigmentation; (b) which responded well to therapy with a Q-switch ruby laser.

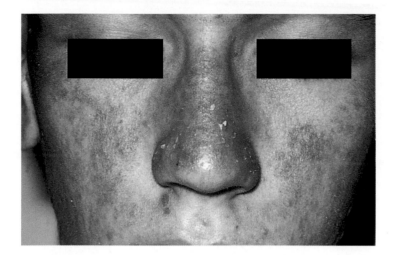

Figure 9.9

Patient with phototoxicity associated with doxycycline therapy.

Interaction with the oral contraceptive

A frequently debated side-effect is the possible effect oral antibiotics may have on reducing the function of the contraceptive pill, a factor that the authors should discuss with their patients. The authors recommend additional physical methods of contraception, especially in the first month of coprescribed therapy, and where it is available recommend Dianette®.

Hormonal therapies

Hormonal therapies are indicated in females responding well to conventional therapy and in women who required oral acne therapy and oral contraception.

There are three major types of hormonal therapy:

1   Oestrogen + cyproterone acetate (Dianette®)
2   Oestrogen + chlormadinonacetate (Belara®)
3   Spironolactone

In Europe, Asia and Australasia Dianette® is available on prescription. It is a combination of 35 mg ethinylestradiol and 2 mg cyproterone acetate. This treatment is usually excellent therapy for the female who requires contraception, period regulation and has acne requiring oral antibiotics. Chlormadinonacetate (CMA) plus ethinylestradiol is available in several European countries, both CPA and CMA, are also available as monodrug formulations. Currently mini-pills with dienogest as an anti-androgen have been released to the market.

As with oral antibiotics the rate of response is slow. There will be no response within the first month and sometimes very little in 6 weeks. Patients who respond less well can be given 50–100 mg cyproterone acetate from days 5–14 of the menstrual cycle.

In older patients, especially in those over the age of 30 years with absolute or relative contraindications to the contraceptive pill, there is some virtue in the use of spironolactone, 100–200 mg/day. The response is dose-dependent and as with other hormonal regimes, spironolactone should be given for 6–36 months in addition to topical therapy. Estradiolvalerate plus 1 mg CPA (Climen®) is also available as an alternative in the elderly acne female patient. Recently an oral contraceptive containing 0.035 mg of ethinylestradiol combined with noregestimate was demonstrated as effective in moderate acne vulgaris. From the experience of European dermatology however, this combination is to be expected less effective as those pills containing cyproterone acetate or chlormadinone acetate available in most countries of the world.

Mechanism of action of hormonal therapy

The precise mechanism of action of the hormonal regimes is not entirely certain but both systemic and local modulation of hormonal production and hormonal action occurs. There is often a reduction in plasma levels of testosterone and dehydroepiandrostenedione and, more recently, it has been shown that they reduce the conversion of androgens by sebocytes and probably also in follicular keratinocytes. The overall effect of cyproterone acetate is a dose-dependent reduction in sebum excretion and an effect on comedogenesis (Figure 9.10). The estrogen

part of the combination pills increases SHBG, which can consequently bind more free testosterone.

Side-effects of hormonal therapy

In general, they are no different to those seen with other contraceptives, except that Dianette® is more likely to produce weight gain. Six-monthly checks of blood pressure and breasts are necessary and cervical smears should be examined every 2–3 years depending on local regulations.

Spironolactone is not a contraceptive and this must be emphasized to the patient. Its main side-effects are hormonal in nature, in particular menstrual irregularities. Fifteen per cent of the patients cannot tolerate spironolactone therapy although a reduction in dose may allow continuation of the therapy. There is some controversy about spironolactone promoting breast tumours and leukaemia in animals but there is no human evidence to support this data.

Oral isotretinoin

Oral isotretinoin (13–cis-retinoic acid) therapy has been an important advance in the treatment of patients, initially for those with severe acne, but more recently in those patients with less severe disease.

Clinical indications

There are several indications for the use of oral isotretinoin:

- Severe acne (Figure 9.11)
- Patients with moderate disease who have failed two or three courses of adequate

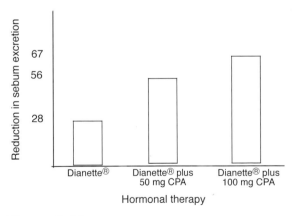

Figure 9.10

The effect of Dianette® alone and Dianette® plus 50 or 100 mg cyproterone acetate (CPA) on sebum excretion.

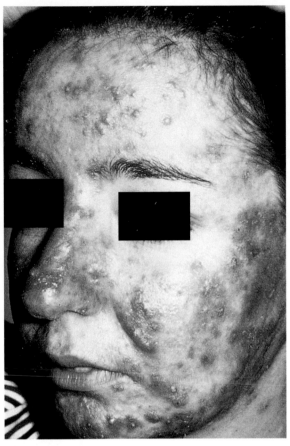

Figure 9.11

A patient with severe acne who clearly needs oral isotretinoin therapy because of the high risk of significant scarring.

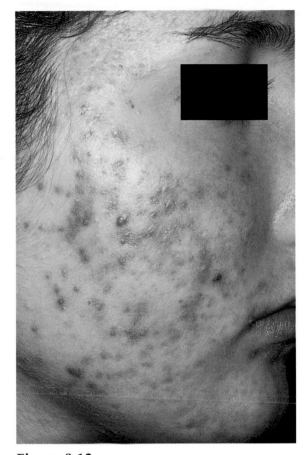

Figure 9.12

This patient who failed to respond to two or three courses of adequate conventional therapy was then prescribed oral isotretinoin.

conventional therapy (Figure 9.12). Just how long physicians describe adequate conventional therapy differs. In the authors' practice it is usually a total of 6–12 months of such therapy, whereas, in other clinics it is a total of 6 months. In the authors' clinics rarely is oral isotretinoin prescribed without having prescribed 200 mg minocycline and sometimes also 600 mg trimethoprim. Some physicians will prescribe oral isotretinoin having only prescribed 100 mg minocycline

- Patients with significant scarring independent of the severity of acne, who are still developing acne lesions and scarring from the acne
- Patients with significant psychosocial distress from the disease independent of the degree of acne. There is a need to use such psychosocial forms in the clinic to allow the detection of psychosocial problems as well as to detect potential drug-related depressive effects of isotretinoin.

Acne variants can also be treated with oral isotretinoin, in particular:

- Gram-negative folliculitis
- Acne fulminans
- Pyoderma faciale (rosacea fulminans).

In the two latter conditions, oral isotretinoin should not be given until oral steroids have been prescribed for 4–6 weeks, otherwise there could be a tremendous flare of the patient's cutaneous and systemic features (Figure 9.13). The recommended dose of oral prednisolone is 0.5–1.0 mg/kg and the dose of oral steroids can be reduced as the dosage of the oral isotretinoin is gradually introduced.

Dose regimes

Although there have been many studies, no very large evidence-based conclusive studies have indicated precisely which patients should receive what dose. Often the dose regime given by the physician is based on his or her own experience.

Many physicians usually start the patient on a dose somewhere between 0.5–1.0 mg/kg, rarely higher. Patients with severe acne, younger males and those with truncal acne may begin with a 1.0 mg/kg dose regime, but other patients often start on the lower dose of 0.5 mg/kg. It could be argued that, since the side-effects are dose-dependent, there is some justification in starting with the lower dose of 0.5 mg/kg and gradually building the dose up to a level of maximum tolerance, which is usually 1.0 mg/kg. Rarely is there any justification for using doses of greater than 1.0 mg/kg.

Duration of therapy

Most patients will receive 4–6 months of therapy. The duration of therapy is at times related to the physician's understanding of the term 'cumulative' dose. This refers to how much oral isotretinoin the patient receives throughout a course. Evidence from Saurats' group in Geneva suggests that there is no justification in giving doses beyond 120 mg/kg. Only exceptionally is it necessary to prolong the course of oral isotretinoin beyond this cumulative dose. If indeed this is necessary, the authors suggest that the patient should be classed as a poor responder, for which there are several explanations.

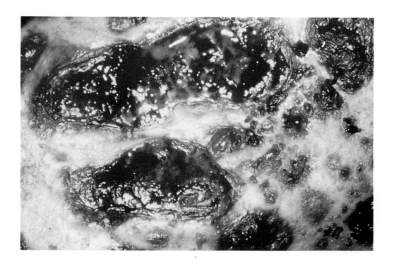

Figure 9.13

A patient with acne fulminans in whom oral steroids should be given before starting oral isotretinoin therapy.

Relapse post-isotretinoin therapy

Current data suggests that relapse post-isotretinoin therapy is 30–40%, thus, 60–70% of subjects will probably need no oral isotretinoin again. Some, however, may require oral antibiotics, but usually either no treatment or just topical therapy. The reason for the long-term benefit of oral isotretinoin, months or years after stopping therapy, is unknown.

Reasons for poor response to oral isotretinoin

Macrocomedones

Macrocomedones (Figure 9.14) can be a focus of a severe acne flare. This is likely to be secondary to a reduction in the sebum excretion resulting in the death of many *P. acnes* organisms and consequent release of many inflammatory antigens, which can trigger the horrendous flares of acne.

Since significant scarring may result, such patients should have their macrocomedones treated with gentle cautery, prior to oral isotretinoin therapy.

If problems are detected while on therapy, then oral isotretinoin should be stopped or the dose reduced to a small dose such as 10 mg/day. The dose can subsequently be increased after the physical therapy (cautery) of their macrocomedones. Oral steroids (0.5 mg/kg) for 3–4 weeks are also usually necessary.

Severe nodular acne

Severe nodular acne can be associated with slow progress, simply because the lesions are so intensely inflammatory or initially beyond redemption in terms of responding to oral isotretinoin. Oral steroids (e.g. prednisolone 0.5–1.0 mg/kg/day), intra-lesional steroids (e.g. triamcinalone) or dexamethasone cream applied twice daily to big papules for 7 days may be required. These physical methods of therapy are described in Chapter 10.

Slow responding disease

There is a group of patients who do not respond well for reasons that are not obvious.

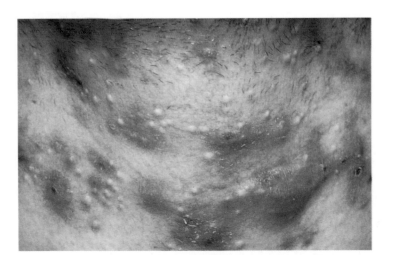

Figure 9.14

Patient with many macrocomedones, which flared into troublesome inflammatory lesions when treated with oral istotretinoin.

In such patients, it may be necessary to continue therapy for longer than 6 months.

Side-effects

For a discussion of the side-effects see later.

Poor absorption of isotretinoin

Some patients cannot absorb isotretinoin readily and thus respond poorly to treatment. The authors have had the opportunity of investigating a few patients, especially those who are on multiple therapies who have not developed the clinical benefit and side-effects associated with oral isotretinoin. Measurement of their sebum excretion has shown it not to be greatly suppressed. In such patients it is worthy of increasing the dose to 1.5–2.0 mg/kg or in exceptional cases to 3.0 mg/kg/day.

Repeat courses of oral isotretinoin

Patients frequently ask if repeat courses of oral isotretinoin can be given. They can and the usual principles for prescribing oral isotretinoin are required. Response is predictable, the outcome similar and some patients have required five or six courses of oral isotretinoin over 18 years, but this is unusual.

Intermittent dosage for sebosuppression

In a small number of patients the acne is sufficiently controlled, but seborrhoea is still severe. In this case, we recommend a 2–3 times weekly dose of 20–30 mg/day.

Side-effects of oral isotretinoin

Oral isotretinoin is a drug with many side-effects, that is why it should be reserved until other treatments have failed or until the scarring and psychosocial problems of the patient are such that urgent treatment with oral isotretinoin is a must. The side-effects can be divided into mucocutaneous and systemic side-effects. Table 9.1 lists the common and uncommon mucocutaneous side-effects.

Table 9.1   Mucocutaneous side-effects of isotretinoin.

Common side-effects	Incidence (%)
Cheilitis (Figure 9.15)	95
Facial erythema	67
Facial dermatitis	65
Vestibulitis/epistaxis (Figure 9.16)	55
Blepharoconjunctivitis	30
Primary irritant dermatitis (Figure 9.17)	
Discoid eczema	30 (cumulative)
Follicular eczema	
Xeroderma	

Uncommon side-effects	Incidence (%)
Impetiginized eczema (Figure 9.18)	7
Boils (Figure 9.19)	3
Acne flare	2
Paronychia	2
Scalp folliculitis	2
Skin fragility	2
Pyogenic granulomata (Figure 9.20)	1
Sun sensitivity	1
Hair loss	0.5
Curly hair (Figure 9.21)	0
Eruptive xanthomata	0
Osteoma cutis	0
Erythema nodosum	0

The last four entries (Curly hair, Eruptive xanthomata, Osteoma cutis, Erythema nodosum) are bracketed together as <0.1%.

Common mucocutaneous side-effects can be treated by:

- Reduction in dose of isotretinoin
- Regular use of moisturisers, including lipsalves, three or four times daily even in the first few days of therapy
- If necessary, a medium-strength topical corticosteroid ointment
- If there is any hint of infection (the skin colonizes with *S. aureus* easily while on oral isotretinoin), a topical antimicrobial agent such as pseudomonic acid may be required. If a topical steroid is required, it can be combined with a topical antiseptic cream (e.g. clioquinol) and oral antistaphylococcal therapy (i.e. flucloxacillin).

Uncommon side-effects are treated by dose-reduction and by symptomatic relief as highlighted in more extensive texts.

Oral side-effects of isotretinoin

The most important oral side-effect of isotretinoin is teratogenicity. It is essential that a female to be prescribed oral isotretinoin must be using adequate contraceptive measures 1 month before starting treatment, while on treatment and for 6 weeks after stopping therapy. A pregnancy test is necessary 2–3 days before starting therapy and the physician should see the patient just about the time of her period and the drug started on the second or third day of the period. Some physicians insist on the oral contraceptive pill. It is the responsibility of female patients to decide upon the best method, but it is important for the physician to discuss the issue fully with them. The authors insist that the patient signs a document indicating that all these issues have been discussed. There are many other systemic side-effects listed in Table 9.2. The most common of these are:

Table 9.2 Systemic side-effects of oral isotretinoin.

Side-effects	Incidence (%)
Teratogenicity	100 nsn therapy
Myalgia	
Arthralgia	30–40
Headaches	
Night blindness*	
Opticatrophy*	
Optic neuritis*	
Mood swings*	
Depression*	<2%
Hepatitis*	
Tinnitus*	
Diffuse interstitial hyperostosis* (Figure 9.22)	

*Often much less.

- Headaches: these may normally respond to dose reduction, or paracetamol, panadol or an NSAID such as ibuprofen.
- Arthralgias and myalgias: these occur particularly in more athletic individuals and, like headaches, need little (paracetamol or ibuprofen may be required) or no treatment. Dose reduction may also be necessary.

Other less common systemic side-effects are highlighted in Table 9.2, but, of these, the most significant are mood changes and depression.

With regard to mood changes and depression: oral isotretinoin improves dramatically the psychosocial well-being of patients with acne. In a few patients, however, drug-induced mood swings and depression occur. It may be difficult to detect the latter as the depression may not present typically, instead patients may be agitated or violent; if not looked for specifically it can be missed.

There is a need for a large prospective study to compare acne scarring to acne severity, and drug-related issues to disease-related issues. In the interim it is important that all physicians discuss these issues with the patients. Ideally, the facts should be shared with their family.

In the authors' clinics patients are asked to sign a note indicating that these issues have been discussed with the patient. In addition, the Roche data sheet must be given to the patient some days before starting therapy.

In Appendix I is listed patient documentation used in the authors' clinics to ensure that the relevant issues have been discussed with patients and, if necessary, their

relatives. Included there is a summary of the side-effects given to all patients highlighting the more relevant features of their treatment.

Other oral therapies

There have been many publications on the potential benefit of other oral therapies, usually before the advent of oral isotretinoin. These include clofazimine, dapsone, oral

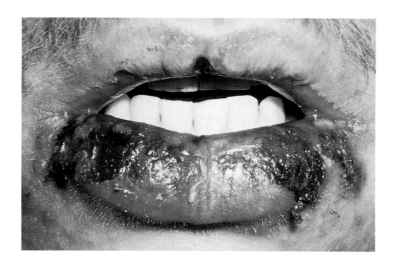

Figure 9.15

Typical severe cheilitis in a patient taking oral isotretinoin.

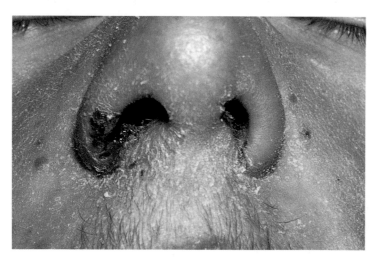

Figure 9.16

Typical severe nasal crusting in a patient taking oral isotretinoin.

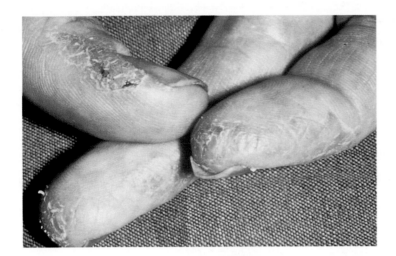

Figure 9.17

Typical irritant dermatitis of the hands in a patient taking oral isotretinoin.

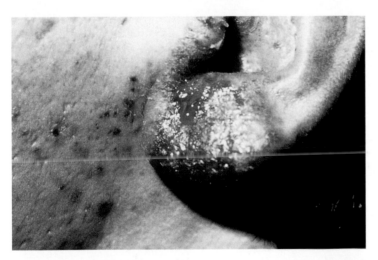

Figure 9.18

Impetiginized eczema in a patient taking oral isotretinoin.

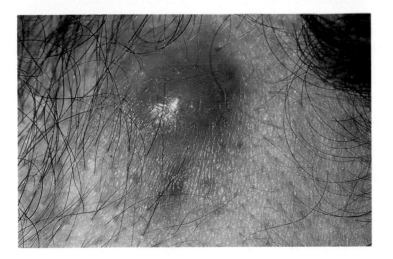

Figure 9.19

Typical boils in a patient taking oral isotretinoin.

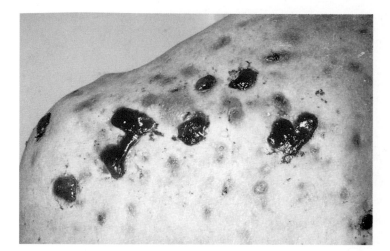

Figure 9.20

Pyogenic granuloma in a patient taking oral isotretinoin.

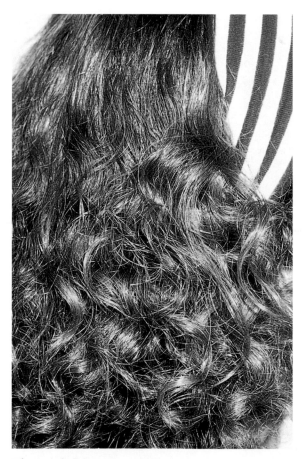

Figure 9.21

Curly hair in a patient taking oral isotretinoin.

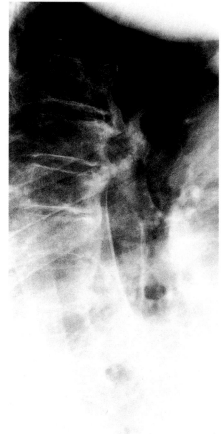

Figure 9.22

Diffuse interstitial hyperostosis showing typical calcification of the anteriovertebral ligaments.

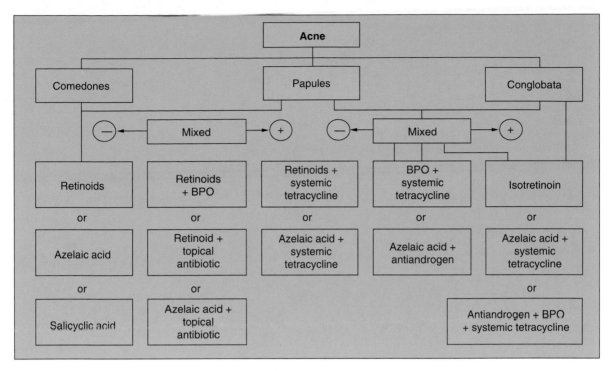

Figure 9.23

General scheme to help decide which and when topical and oral therapy should be used.

steroids, non-steroidal anti-inflammatory agents (NSAIDs), zinc, antidepressants and anxiolytic drugs.

Dapsone has been shown to have virtually little or no effect. Oral steroids are certainly of benefit in patients with late-onset adrenal hyperplasia (5 mg/day preferably taken at night). Moreover, oral steroids are of immense value in a patient who presents with or develops atrocious inflammatory acne; 0.5–1.0 mg/kg/day for 2 weeks, reducing to zero over 4 weeks, which can dramatically reduce the degree of inflammation. Oral steroids are also required in patients with acne fulminans and pyoderma faciale before isotretinoin is prescribed. Although NSAIDs have been shown to be beneficial in combination with oral antibiotics they are not widely prescribed.

The patient who is unquestionably depressed or anxious because of his acne may require appropriate psychotherapeutic drugs as well as counselling. If necessary, referral to a psychiatrist may then be essential.

10 Physical treatment of active acne and of acne scarring

Introduction

Physical treatments for acne are occasionally used but less then other therapies since on the whole they are less effective.

Physical treatment of inflammatory acne

Intralesional triamcinolone

Intralesional triamcinolone acetonide can be particularly helpful in the treatment of large nodules, particularly if they have been present for 7 days or less. This may be best preceded by using a wide-bore needle to aspirate from the bottom of such nodules semi-solid inflammatory material. It is also useful to allow drainage of what is a multi-locular lesion before injecting the triamcinilone. Gentle pressure down towards the orifice of the iatrogenically produced hole may increase the drainage of this semipurulent material. It is then best to inject the triamcinolone into the upper part of the nodular lesion to avoid it simply running out through the hole. Gentle massage of the lesion allows the steroids to diffuse into the nodule. The amount injected varies but is usually around 0.1–0.2 ml. The typical concentration of triamcinilone used is either 20 mg or 40 mg/ml. It is important not to inject the steroid near the eyes, since, rarely, this has entered the ocular apparatus and produced blindness. Repeat injections in the same cyst can be given on two occasions over 10 days if necessary; this is best avoided, however, because of the potential atrophic effect of the injected steroid.

Cryotherapy

Inflammatory nodular lesions that have been present beyond 7 days may be treated with cryotherapy: 5–20 seconds over 1 full cycle. Surprisingly, this is relatively more pain-free than the physician and patient may imagine; pre-operatively, however, simple analgesia such as paracetamol can be prescribed if necessary. Very occasionally blistering may arise at the site of cryotherapy which can be treated by the patient. After wiping the skin with an alcohol soap swab, patients gently prick the skin with a small needle to allow drainage of any seropurulent material. The purpose of this treatment is to encourage the body's own defence mechanisms to eradicate the rather static nodular lesion. Histology following such therapy shows that, within a few days, many polymorphs accumulate in the nodule.

Physical treatment of comedones

A comedone extractor may be used. Regrettably, however, the design of many comedone extractors makes physical treatment more difficult on areas of soft skin that do not lay over a prominent bone. Thus areas over the zygoma and the forehead are much easier to treat than in the middle of the cheek.

Gentle cautery of macrocomedones

This is discussed on page 125 to which the reader is referred.

Physical treatment of scars

The various clinical types of acne scarring are discussed in Chapter 5.

It is important to stress that acne scars are not so easily treated as inflammatory and comedonal acne. It is important to have several interviews with the patient before starting any procedure, which may be time-consuming, uncomfortable and possibly produce an unsatisfactory outcome. It is thus most important to ascertain the psychosocial impact that the scarring has on the patient and to make sure that the patient's expectations are not unrealistic.

Owing to the very high technical standard required by many of the techniques it is recommended that an experienced dermatologist performs the procedure.

The objective of all rehabilitative procedures is to achieve an acceptable physical appearance of the surface of the facial skin and other acne prone areas. In some patients, several procedures may be required.

Treatment of ice-pick and atrophic scars

Bovine collagen injections

Bovine collagen injections may be useful in the treatment of superficial ice-pick scars and in atrophic scars. A prerequisite is that the scar to be treated can be easily stretched and ideally have only little or no fibrosis. Deep ice-pick scars with a fibrotic base and keloids do not benefit from such injections.

If bovine collagen injections are to be considered, it is necessary to determine that patients or family members do not have a history of autoimmune disease or of any history of granulomatous disease.

If there are no contraindications, a test dose of the bovine collagen is performed intradermally on the forearm to exclude a hypersensitive reaction to the collagen. The injected site is reviewed at 3–6 weeks. If the test is negative (a positive reaction has an incidence of about 1%) then the bovine collagen can be injected into the scars to overcorrect the scar deficiency by one-and-a-half of the amount estimated to fill the dermal defect. Depending on the area, in particular in the face, local pain may occur at the time of the injection. Often two or three injections are given at monthly intervals.

The bovine collagen injection not only replaces the collagen, but electron microscopy studies have shown it to be replaced by human collagen.

The bovine collagen types that are frequently used are the Zyderm 1™ (35 mg/ml), the Zyderm II™ (65 mg/ml) and the Zyplast™ (75 mg/ml).

Side-effects include a granulomatous reaction despite a negative intradermal test.

Autologous fat replacement

The autologous material is obtained by aspiration with a needle from, for example, the girdle area, homogenized and the atrophic scar filled in the same way as with the bovine collagen at least with one and a half to one fold overfill of the amount to be replaced. This procedure has to be performed under sterile conditions. It is possible to store the patient's fat in order to re-treat the same or other areas at a later date.

Punch biopsy elevation

Small fibrotic and non-fibrotic depressed scars can be elevated using a punch biopsy. The results are better in non-fibrotic scars. The scarplug is raised to the level of the surrounding skin niveau and either fixed by a no. 6.0 suture or by fibrin adhesive or an adhesive tape. Sutures have to be removed early to prevent scarring and tunnel formation.

Punch excision with full-thickness graft replacement

This method is useful in treating fibrotic scars in which elevation alone is not possible. The punch has to be fixed by a fibrin adhesive or an adhesive tape. The donor site should have a facial skin-like pattern of adnexae to prevent a strange recipient site appearance.

Electrodesiccation

Electrodesiccation has its place in adapting the shadow-casting edges of small crateriform acne scars. Usually the electrodesiccation technique is combined with punch biopsy elevation.

Excision of draining sinuses (black type)

In the more severe forms of acne, draining sinuses can occur in the face and, in particular, genital and axillary regions. If the sinuses are shorter than 1 cm in length they can be incised and drained. Larger ones should be excised and allowed to heal by forming granulation tissue. Sinus disease is best treated when the sinus tract is not inflamed. A course of oral steroids or potent topical steroids applied, albeit only for 7–10 days may help to settle any persistent, non-acute inflammation. Sadly, significant scarring is often seen following such surgery.

Dermabrasion

Dermabrasion is a method usually performed under general anaesthesia but some smaller areas can be treated under local anaesthesia. This technique requires excellent training, and considerable experience, since dermabrasion performed too superficially will be disappointing for the patient and the physician, and if performed too deeply, widespread scarring and hyper- and/or hypopigmentation can occur. The aim of dermabrasion is to level off superficial scars and to minimize deep and atrophic scars. It is particularly helpful in ice-pick and atrophic scars that are characterized by crateriform lesions, which give irregular and multiple shadows to the skin. Dermabrasion reduces the contrast. Some patients with ice-pick scars have a bottle-shaped scar that is narrower nearer the surface, the deeper part of the scar being wider. In such patients, dermabrasion may lead to unsuccessful results by making the scars more noticeable than pre-surgery.

It is beyond the aims of this booklet to provide in depth details of this procedure, which is now performed much less than it was since the advent of carbon dioxide (CO_2) laserbrasion.

Post-inflammatory hyperpigmentation may occur with dermabrasion; this can be controlled by the patient staying out of the sunshine for at least 1 month and with adequate use of sunblocks. Conversely, hypopigmentation may occur. A further complication is herpes simplex, which can be prevented with prophylactic oral acyclovir.

Cryopeeling

Cryopeeling represents a superficial freezing of diseased skin. It is indicated only in very small but widespread hypertrophic scars, particularly on the face and in patients without inflammatory acne lesions. A 2×2 cm cryoprobe is applied to the skin for some seconds until a very thin frost occurs. When this occurs, the probe is immediately moved to the next area until the whole of the affected skin area has been frozen. Usually this method is limited to the facial skin and has to follow exactly the tension lines. Erythema occurs for 1–3 days and this is followed by a superficial desquamation.

The treatment is repeated every 4 weeks until a satisfying result is achieved (sometimes, however, results are not very good). As with dermabrasion, the procedure is best performed in winter to avoid post-inflammatory hyperpigmentation.

Laserdermablation

Depending on the type of scars, different lasers come into use. In hypertrophic scars which still show increased vascularization both a vessel-directed or a fibrous tissue-destroying laser type can be used. Flashlamp pumped pulsed dye laser (FLPDL) has been reported to be very effective. Several sessions are necessary, 5–7 J/cm²/5 mm or 4.5–6.25 J/cm²/7 mm dose and diameter can be used.

All lasers that work by ablation induce superficial scarring. Carbon dioxide (CO_2) or erbium YAG-lasers are used today. In principle, there is evidence that those patients prone to develop hypertrophic scars and keloids are in the situation to respond with new scarring. For prophylaxis of relapse of scarring local pressure by specially made clothes can be used. In addition, cryotherapy can be used in combination and/or additional topical glucocorticosteroid tapes can be applied. The steroid can also be injected.

In keloids which are not particularly inflamed, the flash pump dye laser is not indicated, but the CO_2-laser is. The CO_2-laser should be used in the vaporizing mode followed by cryotherapy in the same session. This is followed by compression. Widespread superficial atrophic acne scarring is a good indication also for laser ablation. In contrast to the use of the laser types in aged skin no collagen shrinking is wanted. The authors prefer to use the erbium YAG-laser or the CO_2-laser with flash scanner. It is important that the laser is used in complete anatomical skin areas such as the perioral region, cheeks, chin or forehead. Treatment of circumscribed areas usually leads to disappointing results with erythema, hyper- and hypopigmentation with a mottling appearance. The clinical results are quite satisfying with some physicians reporting up to 80% improvement for example with the pulsed CO_2-laser.

Chemical peeling

Chemical peeling has gained increasing popularity particularly in the private clinical practice in most European countries. However, depending on the type of chemical peeling methods used, some have to be performed in an inpatient situation. In general, this method is used in superficial scarring. The peeling substances are α-hydroxy acetic acids (glycolic acid), trichloroacetic acid, dichloroacetic acid and zinc chloride. There are many protocols involved in different combinations of chemicals, some are also used in combination with laser dermablation. Usually, one starts with a 2-week course of 10–15% glycolic acid, daily application, then increasing the concentration up to 20–35% weekly or every second week. To induce better and deeper effects one has to use concentrations up to 70%. The application time until the neutralization of the pH can also be increased. The glycolic acid concentrations, time of application and interval between therapies can be adapted to the patient's individual need; deeper effects can be obtained by 20% TCA in water, concentrations up to 45% are also in use. The application of phenolum liquefactum is no longer recommended by the authors.

Contraindications for chemical peeling

Those patients not closely cooperating with the physician should not be treated. There is evidence that patients should be off oral isotretinoin for 1 year. Frequently relapsing herpes simplex is a relative contraindication. However, occasional herpes simplex infection is an absolute contraindication and prophylactic acyclovir can be prescribed. Peeling should normally not be performed during the sunny time of the year. This booklet is not aimed at giving precise practical details. The more significant peeling methods are reserved for the very experienced dermatologist but good evidence-based medicine is lacking.

Treatment of hypertrophic scars and keloids

The treatment of this type of scarring in acne is not very successful, however, some improvement may be achieved but control studies are lacking. There are different modalities of treatment, which comprises topical and intralesional corticosteroids, swift-CO_2-laser ablation, cryotherapy and silicone plaster.

Hypertrophic scars can be treated by application of fluorinated corticosteroid creams either with or without occlusion overnight for up to 2 months. To avoid atrophy of normal skin, great care has to be taken not to apply the corticosteroid to the surrounding normal skin. If there is no response to therapy after 2 months, the steroid triamcinolone acetonide (5 mg/ml) can be injected at 3-weekly intervals on two or three occasions (0.1–0.3 ml depending on the size of the scar). Normally, a local anaesthetic is not required. The injection will usually help the itching if this is a feature. Unfortunately, there is a recurrence rate of 50% following such therapies.

In patients in which the injection is painful owing to firmness of the keloid, a topical anaesthetic such as EMLA® cream can be applied at least 45 minutes before injection. An alternative approach is to ablate the hypertrophic scar using a swift CO_2 laser immediately followed by cryotherapy contact freezing. Some physicians also inject triamcinolone into the base of the 'removed' keloid. Limited evidence supports the view that combination therapies give the best results.

Less painful options include long-term treatment with topical tretinoin 0.05% solution for up to 3 months; other alternatives include superficial X-rays. Topical application of silicone gel dressings which have to be applied for several days to the keloid or hypertrophic scar and to a few millimetres of the surrounding normal skin.

After 3 months, a flattening of lesions has been reported.

Newer experimental modalities include the intralesional injection of recombinant interferon-γ (0.01 mg, three times/week), which can lead to a significant reduction in the size of the keloids after three weeks. Intralesional injections of superoxide dismutase or hyaluronidase did not show better results than interlesional corticosteroid injections.

In very large keloids, particularly located over the shoulder and afflicting more than 30 × 30 cm, local pressure by specially made garments worn for at least 4–12 months may help.

In conclusion, controlled studies on the optimum treatment for scars do not exist. There seems to be no published data outlining the normal process of scar resolution. It is clear from the text that the physician has many options (used alone or in combination) to treat many kinds of scars in several ways. One therapeutic option is to do absolutely nothing if the patient has accepted the problem. Perhaps the most successful technique overall in some patients was dermabrasion; this has almost universally been replaced by CO_2 laserbrasion. In the mature patient, facial lifts certainly help the patient with many atrophic scars, especially if associated with lax facial skin.

11 Patients who respond poorly to therapy

Introduction

Despite the availability of many oral and topical therapies for acne, some patients still respond less than ideally and may therefore scar. The purpose of this chapter is to outline the major reasons for a poor response. These include:

- Wrong diagnosis
- Inadequate physical assessment of the patient by the physician
- Inadequate psychological assessment of the patient
- Inadequate assessment of cosmetics and drugs
- Inadequate compliance
- Side-effects of therapy
- *P. acnes* resistance and drug delivery problems
- Inappropriate use of isotretinoin
- Acne variants
- Failure to manage nodular lesions adequately
- Sinus disease
- Inadequate follicular drug concentration.

Wrong diagnosis

Rarely is this the explanation for a patient's poor response to therapy. The reader is referred to Chapter 6, in which is discussed the differential diagnosis of acne. In particular, confusion may arise with dental sinuses, sebaceous gland hyperplasia, rosacea and human immunodeficiency virus (HIV) eosinophilic folliculitis or overlying staphylococcal or Gram-negative infection.

Inadequate physical assessment of the patient by the physician

No physician would treat hypertension without monitoring blood pressure, nor would a diabetologist control diabetes without knowing blood sugar levels. Despite the accessibility of the skin, many dermatologists are not good at assessing acne. The clinical examination can be performed quite easily in the clinic provided the physician has good light. The assessment can be made on a global scheme using one of several techniques now available (see Chapter 5). The former technique is quick, taking but a few minutes.

The choice of topical therapy should not be made without examining the skin using a good light and a ×4 lens, without which the presence of many whiteheads will be missed (see Chapter 5). Stretching of the skin is mandatory to highlight their presence. The presence of many comedones requires the use of a topical retinoid.

- Assessment of the acne severity will provide better clinical audit
- Adequate assessment of the lesion type with a good light is essential, especially not to miss comedones

---

Inadequate psychological assessment of the patient

Several authors have now produced a whole range of disability indices. The authors use their own questionnaire (15 questions) to better understand how the patient is affected by his or her acne (Appendix B). The maximum score in our system is 144; if a patient achieves a score of 80 or more then it is very clear that the acne is greatly affecting their life. Although there is some correlation between the physical severity of acne and the disability score there is not always a consistent trend. Some patients, especially those for whom the interview takes a long time, have a very high score and yet minimal acne on physical examination. These patients need to be treated with considerable care and attention by both the dermatologist and liaison psychiatrist.

- A measurement of the psychological effect is essential before and durin therapy.

Patient compliance

Inadequate patient compliance is a recognized problem in some patients with chronic disease, be it systemic disease or skin disease; however, lack of compliance is not always perceived by the physician as a reason for a poor response to therapy. Using a phenobarbitone tracer technique the authors have shown that one third of their patients taking either oral minocycline or oral tetracycline fail to take therapy adequately. Some physicians are not aware of the simple clinical observation that some patients with truncal acne do not adequately apply topical therapy to that site. The physician must therefore:

- Stress the need for compliance
- Provide adequate information sheets
- Provide adequate information for the parents in the young acne patient

Side-effects

Failure to recognize or prevent side-effects will influence response to therapy. Some uncommon side-effects may not be recognized easily because they are unusual. The reader is referred to Chapters 8 and 9 for relevant information.

P. acnes resistance

There is increasing evidence to incriminate *Propionibacterium acnes* as a central factor in the development of inflammation. The evidence for this is two-fold: there is a correlation between reduction in *P. acnes* colonization and a clinical improvement. Secondly, in some patients there is an association of

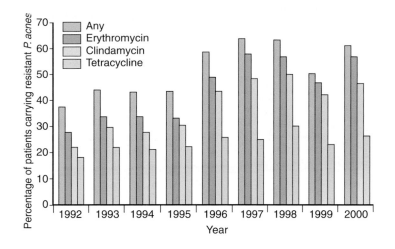

Figure 11.1

Variation in *P. acnes* resistance with time. The figure shows the resistance with different antibiotics.

P. acnes resistance with failure to respond clinically to the antibiotic to which the *P. acnes* is resistant.

In the early 1980s *P. acnes* resistance was unusual; however, there has been a marked increase in *P. acnes* resistance; in the Leeds General Infirmary it is now 69% (Figure 11.1).

P. acnes micro-organisms are not that difficult to grow but few laboratories grow them regularly. The following clinical situations should alert the physician to the likelihood of *P. acnes* resistance.

• Failure to respond despite what is otherwise effective antimicrobial therapy
• Loss of clinical benefit while on therapy
• Long-term oral use of erythromycin
• Use of many different oral and topical antibiotics.

Benzoyl peroxide is not just a useful therapy in both inflammatory and non-inflammatory acne, but it also reduces *P. acnes* resistance. This has been shown particularly in the laboratory. A topical preparation containing 5% benzoyl peroxide and 3% erythromycin– Benzamycin® has been shown to be better than either therapy alone. Likewise it has been shown that zinc acetate will reduce the number of resistant *P. acnes organisms*. Zinc

acetate itself has antimicrobial actions against *P. acnes*. A combined therapy of erythromycin and zinc acetate is available in the form of Zineryt®.

Thus to minimize *P. acnes* resistance the physician should:

• Minimize the use of rotational antibiotics
• Avoid the use of different antibiotics orally and topically at the same time
• Remember to include in the therapeutic regime benzoyl peroxide, at least intermittently to help reduce *P. acnes* resistance
• Consider combined therapies of benzoyl peroxide, for example with topical erythromycin, or topical zinc with erythromycin or with azelaic acid to reduce *P. acnes* resistance

Inappropriate use of isotretinoin

Most physicians are now familiar with the appropriate use of isotretinoin. The aim of this section is to highlight some important practical issues, all of which are discussed in detail in Chapter 9.

Whom to treat

The following patients should, if appropriate, be considered for treatment with isotretinoin therapy:

- Patients with severe acne, to prevent physical and psychological scarring
- Patients with moderate acne who have failed to respond to what otherwise would normally be adequate conventional therapy (Figure 11.2)

- Patients with a tendency to scar or who are scarring
- Patients who are significantly affected psychologically by the acne

Some patients are slow to respond. Reasons for a slow response include:

- The presence of macrocomedones
- The presence of severe nodular acne (Figure 11.3)

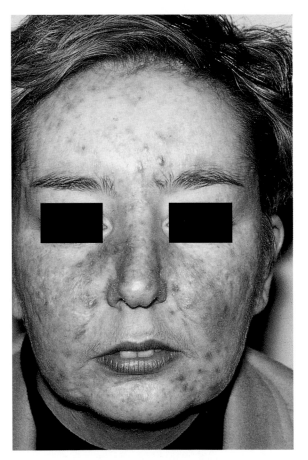

Figure 11.2

Patient with moderate–severe acne who has failed to respond to what would otherwise be adequate conventional treatment. Such patients usually need oral isotretinoin.

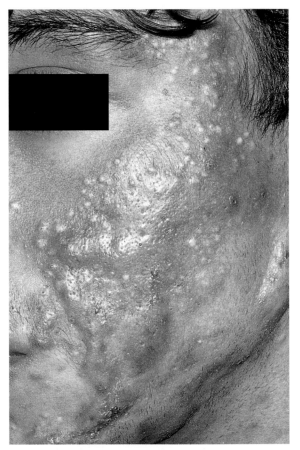

Figure 11.3

Patient with severe nodular acne.

- Endocrine abnormalities, for example polycystic ovaries and congenital adrenal hyperplasia

Relapse

About 60% of patients remain relatively clear of their acne post-therapy but repeat courses of isotretinoin can be given if needed to those who relapse.

Side-effects

Physicians are well aware of the side-effects of isotretinoin. These are discussed in Chapter 9. The major side-effects are:

- Teratogenecity (100% risk)
- Myalgia (common)
- Headaches (common)
- Depression and mood swings (uncommon)
- Mucocutaneous adverse effects (very common)

Pregnancy is contraindicated while on therapy and for 6 weeks post-therapy.

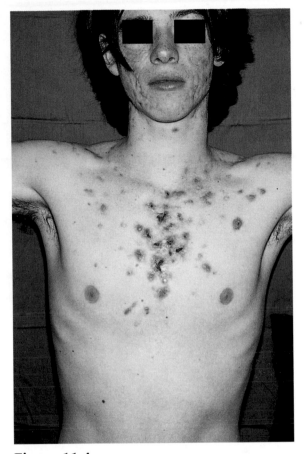

Figure 11.4

Patient with typical acne fulminans.

Severe acne variants

There is a very small percentage of patients with acne that is difficult to treat and these include those with

- Acne conglobata
- Acne fulminans (Figure 11.4)
- Gram-negative folliculitis (Figure 11.5)
- Pyoderma faciale (Rosacea fulminans) (Figure 11.6)
- Hidradenitis suppurativa.

Many of these patients may benefit from isotretinoin therapy but not necessarily as the first line of treatment. These variants are discussed in Chapter 7.

Nodular acne lesions

Therapy of such lesions may comprise:

- Topical application of a potent corticosteroid such as dexamethasone cream, three times a day for five days (Figure 11.7)

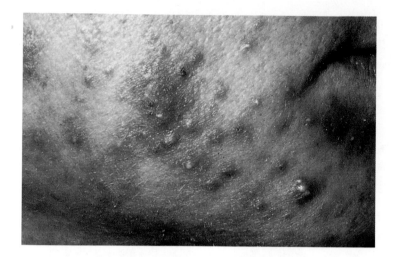

Figure 11.5

Patient with typical Gram-negative folliculitis.

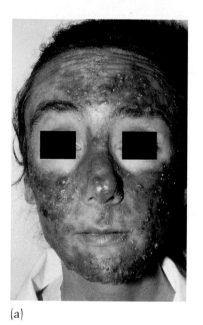

(a)

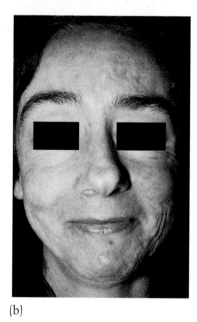

(b)

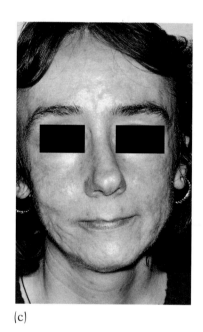

(c)

Figure 11.6

Patient with typical Rosacea fulminans: (a) before, (b) during and (c) after therapy with oral isotretinoin.

- Intralesional triamcinolone: two to three injections over 3–4 weeks
- If the lesion has been present for longer than 3–4 weeks cryotherapy is preferred. Cryotherapy may enhance the rate of resolution by encouraging defence mechanisms to break down perilesional early fibrosis. It is recommended that liquid nitrogen is applied for 10–20 seconds for one or two thaw cycles. Treatment can be repeated 2-weekly

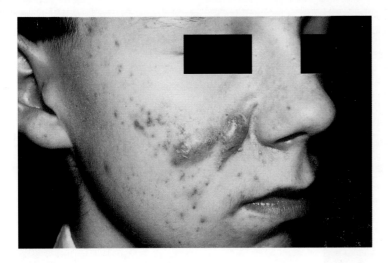

Figure 11.7

Inflammatory sinus tract that might respond a little to potent topical steroids.

Thus treat cysts:

- If acutely inflamed with topical or intralesional steroids
- If less acute with cryotherapy

Sinus disease

Patients with sinus disease (Figures 11.7–11.9) have two or more nodules that are interconnected by epithelial sinus tracts. These are very difficult to treat: response to medical therapies is very varied and perseverance is required with oral antibiotics, oral isotretinoin, topical or intralesional steroids. Incision of acute abscesses may help but this may lead to a more obvious scar than if left. When quiescent, the semi-fibrosed nodules can be removed but often significant scanning is inevitable.

Inadequate follicular drug concentrations

To some extent this relates to resistant *P. acnes*. A lower-than-optimum concentration of an antibiotic in the pilosebaceous unit will encourage the development of *P. acnes* resistance.

Most of the effective antimicrobial therapies for acne have their site of action within the pilosebaceous unit. It is likely that the higher the concentration of the drug the greater the clinical benefit; however, there is no direct evidence for this suggestion since it is as yet impossible to measure follicular levels of anti-acne therapies. There is indirect evidence to support this view since there is a negative correlation between a high sebum excretion and clinical benefit.

However, some patients who do not have *P. acnes* resistance fail to respond to appropriate anti-inflammatory therapies. Such patients often have a high sebum excretion.

This group of patients can be treated in three ways:

1 By increasing the dose of the oral antibiotic. Doses greater than 1 g/day of either tetracycline or oxytetracycline or erythromycin often produce unacceptable side-effects such as abdominal colic, nausea and diarrhoea. Higher doses of doxycycline (150–200 mg/day) are often well tolerated, provided that the doxycycline is taken with much water. Minocycline can be prescribed in doses of 150 mg or 200 mg/day. This is associated with an increased risk of benign

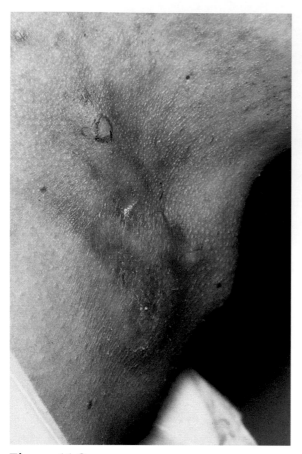

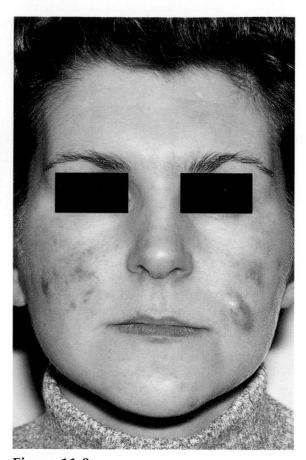

Figure 11.8

Examples of typical sinus disease in which large inflammatory nodules have fused together, resulting in undermining of the skin. In this situation, inflammation rapidly spreads from one nodular lesion to another down the sinus tract.

Figure 11.9

Sinus tract disease.

intracranial hypertension and pigmentation. (This usually occurs in the first 1–3 weeks of therapy.)

2   Female patients who are sexually active have probably been prescribed Dianette®. Such patients can be given, from days 5–14 of their menstrual cycle an additional 50 mg or 100 mg cyproterone acetate for 4–6 months; this will suppress sebum production by a further 50–68%.

3   A third therapeutic regime for such patients is the use of oral isotretinoin.

Conclusion

Most patients with so-called difficult acne should not always be difficult to manage; it is hoped that the issues outlined in this chapter prove to be of help both to the practising physician and to the patient.

Appendices

Appendix A

Standard Acne Therapy Documentation (not Roaccutane)	WQN096

Date: ....

HISTORY

1. Onset of acne: Duration of acne:..............................   Duration of bad acne:...

2. Onset of menarche: Affect of Menses –   No effect ☐ worse ☐ better ☐
                           If worse –   before ☐ during ☐ after ☐
                           Menses *(frequency)*   21–27 ☐ 28–35 ☐ 36–41 ☐ 42+ ☐ days
                           Any recent changes of cycles ....

3. Affect of UVR: No effect ☐ helps   ☐ worsens   ☐ don't know ☐
     Affect of stress   No effect ☐ helps   ☐ worsens   ☐ don't know ☐

PREVIOUS THERAPY

Please note the effect of past therapy, etc: help-H;   No help-NH;   Lost effect-LE;   Don't know-DK; Inadequate therapy-IT.

a. Oral	Daily Dose	Duration	Complied Yes No	Effect		Daily dose	Duration	Complied Yes No	Effect
Aknemin			☐ ☐		Minocycline			☐ ☐	
Dianette			☐ ☐		Minocycline MR			☐ ☐	
Doxycycline			☐ ☐		Oxytetracycline			☐ ☐	
Erythromycin			☐ ☐		Trimethoprim			☐ ☐	
Isotretinoin			☐ ☐		Other			☐ ☐	

b. Topical	Duration	Complied Yes No	Effect		Duration	Complied Yes No	Effect
Adapalene		☐ ☐		Retin A		☐ ☐	
Benzamycin		☐ ☐		Skinoren		☐ ☐	
Benzoyl peroxide		☐ ☐		Steimycin		☐ ☐	
Dalacin T		☐ ☐		Zineryt		☐ ☐	
Isotrex		☐ ☐		Other		☐ ☐	

(c) The Pill – Yes ☐ No ☐   Type:...................... Duration:......................... As a contraception: Yes ☐ No ☐

GENERAL HEALTH

Liver trouble   Yes ☐ No ☐   Kidney trouble Yes ☐ No ☐   Other medication Yes ☐ No ☐
Skin disease   Yes ☐ No ☐   If yes, ...

FAMILY HISTORY OF ACNE

Yes ☐   Age - from .... to ....   Don't know ☐
Mother   Yes ☐ No ☐   Father Yes ☐ No ☐   Brother Yes ☐ No ☐   Sister Yes ☐ No ☐

PSYCHOLOGICAL SCORE (APSEA): ☐ + ☐ + ☐ = ☐
Significance: Appropriate ☐   Low ☐   High ☐   Very high ☐

EXAMINATION

Patient off all therapy for approximately 1 month (except pill)? Yes ☐ No ☐

Grade *(tick)*, **Predominate lesion type, and scar type and grade**

	Acne grade	Superficial inflamed	Deep inflamed	Non-inflamed	Scar (1–5) Grade/type
Face					
Back					
Chest					
Total score					

Scar types *(1–5)*

IPS *(ice pick)* ☐   AM *(atrophic macules)* ☐   PFE *(perifollicular elastolysis)* ☐   H/K *(hypertrophic keloid)* ☐

HIRSUTES – Yes ☐ No ☐   Hidradenitis – Yes ☐ No ☐   And Alopecia – Yes ☐ No ☐

If yes, grade: ....

Abdominal examination: n/e ☐ normal ☐ or not ☐

Tests: *(Tick where appropriate)*

1. Acne swab - face, back, chest
2. Sebum excretion rate
3. Sex hormones (SHBG, Testosterone DHA, Androstenedione. FSH/LH. Prolactin)
4. Ultrasound (for PCO)
5. Biopsy, lesion type
6. Liver function, SGOT & fasting lipids
7. Pregnancy test
8. Others

Follow up in ....weeks to decide treatment.   Letter to GP Yes ☐ No ☐

Date: ....   Today started therapy with *(ring where appropriate)*:

Oral	Dose in mg/day	Oral	Dose in mg/day
1. Aknemin	50, 100, 150, 200 mg	6. Isotretinoin	please transfer to isotretinoin notes
2. Dianette®		7. Minocycline (MR)	50, 100, 150, 200 mg
3. Dianette® + CPA		8. Oxytetracycline	500 mg bd
4. Doxycycline	50, 100, 150, 200 mg	9. Trimethoprim	200 mg bd, 300 mg bd
5. Erythromycin	500 mg bd		

Topical (based on lesion type) bd		
10. Adapalene	14. Dermovate	18. Stiemycin
11. Benzamycin gel	15. Isotrex	19. Zineryt
12. Benzoyl peroxide 5%, 10%	16. Retin A 0.01%, 0.025%, 0.05%	20. Cosmetic advice
13. Dalacin T	17. Skinoren 20%	21. Other

PHYSICAL TREATMENT

1. Cryotherapy ☐
2. Intralesional Triamcinolone +aspiration ☐
3. Macrocomedone therapy ☐
4. Multiple therapy for keloids ☐
5. Others ☐

DATE						
Current therapy						
Complied Yes ☐ No ☐ Effect of therapy*						
Side-effects: *(document)* Oral Yes/No Topical Yes/No Others Yes/No (i.e. Pill)						
Acne grade and acne type –Face –Back –Chest						
Total acne grade:						
Significant scars: Yes/No						
APSEA						
Investigation: –Acne swabs –SER –Others						
Therapy: a) Continue b) Change to (as below-number)						
Follow-up *(weeks)*						

*effect of therapy: worse (W), same (S), bit better (BB), moderately better (MB), excellent (E)

a. Oral

1.	Aknemin	4.	Erythromycin	7.	Minocycline MR	10. Other
2.	Dianette®	5.	Isotretinoin	8.	Oxytetracycline	
3.	Doxycycline	6.	Minocycline	9.	Trimethoprim	

b. Topical

11. Adapalene	14. Dalacin T	17. Skinoren	20. Other
12. Benzamycin	15. Isotrex	18. Steimycin	
13. Benzoyl peroxide	16. Retin A	19. Zineryt	

Appendix B

APSEA (Assessment of the Psycho-Social Effects of Acne)

Date:	Overall clinical grade of acne	☐ Mild ☐ Moderate ☐ Severe
Patient's name:	APSEA score (value)	[ ]
	APSEA score (significance)	☐ Insig. ☐ Low ☐ Med ☐ High ☐ V. High

---

Questions 1 to 6 – please tick (√) the box corresponding to the most appropriate answer

IN THE PAST WEEK

1. Worrying thoughts go through my mind
- ☐ a great deal of the time
- ☐ a lot of the time
- ☐ from time to time, not often
- ☐ only occasionally

2. I can sit at ease and feel relaxed
- ☐ definitely
- ☐ usually
- ☐ not often
- ☐ not at all

3. I feel restless, as if I have to be on the move
- ☐ very much indeed
- ☐ quite a lot
- ☐ not very much
- ☐ not at all

AT THE MOMENT

4. I like what I look like in photographs
- ☐ not at all
- ☐ sometimes
- ☐ very often
- ☐ nearly all the time

5. I wish I looked better
- ☐ not at all
- ☐ sometimes
- ☐ very often
- ☐ nearly all the time

6. On the whole I am satisfied with myself
- ☐ strongly disagree
- ☐ disagree
- ☐ agree
- ☐ strongly agree

Mark each out of 9

Questions 7 to 9 – read the following carefully and put a mark at the point on the line that most accurately represents how you feel, e.g. ⊢─/────

7 I still enjoy the things I used to
Never ⊢────────────────────┤ All the time

8. I am more irritable than usual
Never ⊢────────────────────┤ All the time

9. I feel that I am useful and needed
Never ⊢────────────────────┤ All the time

Questions 10 to 15 – How has your skin condition limited the following activities or made them more difficult or awkward, or less enjoyable since you have had acne – once again, please put a mark at the point on the line, e.g. ⊢─/────

10. Going shopping
Not at all ⊢────────────────────┤ All the time

11. Going out socially to meet friends from outside the home
Not at all ⊢────────────────────┤ All the time

12. Going away for weekends, holidays and outings
Not at all ⊢────────────────────┤ All the time

13. Eating out
Not at all ⊢────────────────────┤ All the time

14. Using public changing rooms/swimming pools
Not at all ⊢────────────────────┤ All the time

15. Do you think your appearance will interfere with your chances of future employment?
Strongly disagree ⊢────────────────────┤ Strongly agree

Mark each out of 10
Note that the higher the score, the greater the problem

Appendix C

Oral Isotretinoin Therapy Documentation	WQN098

Date: ....

DIAGNOSIS: Needs Roaccutane for the following reasons *(ring as required):*

1. Very Severe Acne ☐
2. Rapid Relapser ☐
5. Scarring ☐

3. Partial Responder to Conventional Treatment ☐
4. Primary Psychological Reasons ☐
5. Other ☐

GENERAL HEALTH

	Patient		F/H			Patient		F/H	
	Yes	No	Yes	No		Yes	No	Yes	No
Liver disease	☐	☐	☐	☐	Epileptic	☐	☐	☐	☐
Kidney disease	☐	☐	☐	☐	Psychiatric problems	☐	☐	☐	☐
Cardiovascular disease	☐	☐	☐	☐	Other diseases	☐	☐	☐	☐
					Other medication	☐	☐	☐	☐

Alcohol intake: less than average ☐   average ☐   greater than average ☐

APSEA ☐ + ☐ + ☐ = ▭

Discussions with patient

	side-effects		side-effects
Cheilitis	☐	Nose bleeds	☐
Conjunctivitis	☐	Facial dermatitis	☐
Headaches	☐	Arthralgias	☐
		Other	☐

CONTRACEPTION *(Females only)* ☐   LMP ....
Contraception discussed Yes ☐ No ☐   Method *(tick where appropriate)*
irrelevant ☐   sheath ☐   cap ☐   creams ☐   pill *(specify)* ☐ ....
coil ☐   vasectomy ☐

Doctor .... **has discussed with me the fact that pregnancy is contraindicated whilst I am on the drug Roaccutane and for 6 weeks after stopping the drug. Should I become pregnant during this time I understand that an abortion would be necessary because of the very high risk of damage to a baby conceived during this time. Also discussed with me is the very uncommon risk of significant mood changes, depression and suicide. I have a telephone contact if I am concerned.**

Signed	Witness
Date	Date

Pregnancy Test: Yes ☐ No ☐   Date:...   Pos ☐ Neg ☐

Blood tests ordered: fasting lipids ☐   LFTs and SGOT ☐   Haemoglobin ☐

Normal ☐ or not ☐ *(specify)* ....

DISH X-rays ordered (after multiple courses of Roccutane) *(lateral/dorsal spine and heels)* Yes ☐ No ☐

Acne Grade   Face...................... Back...................... Chest...................... TOTAL ....

Date..

Additional Problems   Gram negative folliculitis ☐   Rosacea ☐

Weight *(kgs)* ....   **Dose given** .... mgs   Roaccutane .... = mgs/kg

Instruction leaflet given Yes ☐ No   Telephone number given Yes ☐ No ☐

Next follow up ....

DATE	PRE-THERAPY			
Weeks on therapy				
Grade:				
Face				
Back				
Chest				
Total				
Effect of therapy*				
Clinical side-effects				
Arthralgia				
Cheilitis				
Conjunctivitis				
Depression/Suicide				
Dermatitis elsewhere				
Facial dermatitis				
Headache				
Malaise				
Mood changes				
Nose-bleeds				
Others				
Laboratory investigations – to order if appropriate, NOTE ABNORMAL RESULT				
LFTs & SGOT				
Lipids *(fasting)*				
APSEA				
X-ray (DISH)				
Swab – nose/lesion				
SER				
Others				
Dose given *(mg/kg, total mg)*				
Other treatments				
i.e. Macrocomedone treatment				
Oral steroid				
Topical steroid				
Contraception stressed				
Follow-up				

effect of therapy: worse(W),   same (S),   bit better (BB),   moderately better (MB),   excellent (E)

Appendix D

Summary instructions for taking oral isotretinoin

1. Please take .... capsules each day at the end of your main meal.

2. Stop all other acne therapy unless specifically told.

3. A lipsalve must be used regularly four to five times per day from the first day of starting the therapy. This can be bought at any chemist.

4. Should the skin become dry, do use a moisturizer.

5. For the occasional headaches or aches and pains take Panadol.

6. Make sure that you have a follow up appointment to see me in eight weeks time.

7. In the case of females, it is VERY IMPORTANT that you DO NOT become pregnant whilst on therapy or for 6 weeks after stopping therapy.

8. Please note the rare side effects of mood swings, depression and suicide.

9. In the sun always use a No. 15 sunblock.

10. Please discuss these issues with your family and friends.

11. Please call the clinic at any time if you have a problem. If in any doubt, insist on speaking to a doctor.

References

Chapter 1

Gollnick H, Zouboulis ChC, Akamatsu H et al, Pathogenesis-related treatment of acne. *J Dermatol* (1991) **18**: 489–499.

Röpke E, Augustin W, Gollnick H, Improved method for studying skin lipid samples from cyanoacrylate strips by high-perforance thin layer chromatography. *Skin Pharmacol* (1996) **9**: 381–387.

Zouboulis ChC, Krieter A, Gollnick H et al, Progressive differentiation of human sebocytes in vitro is charactrized by increasing cell size and altering antigen expression and is regulated by culture duration and reinoids. *Exp Dermatol* (1994) **3**: 151–160.

Chapter 3

Forssman T, Gloor M, Gehring W, Antibiotikaresistenzen bei Acne vulgaris – Eine retrospektive Untersuchung an einem antibiotisch vorbehandelten und einem unbehandelten Kollektiv. *Z Hautkr 69* (1994) **12**: 828–832.

Vogt K, Hermann J, Blume U et al, Comparative activity of a topical quinolone, OPC-7251, against bacteria associated with acne vulgaris. *Eur J Clin Microb Inf Dis* (1992) **11**: 943–945.

Chapter 4

Cunliffe WJ, *Acne*. London: Martin Dunitz (1989) 232–245.

Eady EA, Ingham E, *Propionibacterium acnes* – a friend or foe? *Rev Med Microbiol* (1994) **5**: 163–173.

Ingham E, Eady EA, Goodwin CE et al, Pro-inflammatory levels of interleukin-1α-like bioactivity are present in the majority of open comedones in acne vulgaris. *J Investigative Derm* (1992) **98**: 895–901.

Kligman AM, An overview of acne. *J Investigative Dermatol* (1974) **62**: 268–287.

Layton AM, Morris C, Ingham E, Cunliffe WJ, Immunohistochemical examination of the evolving acne lesion. *J Investigative Dermatol* (1994) **104**: 443.

Leeming JP, Holland KT, Cunliffe WJ, The microbial colonisation of inflamed acne vulgaris lesions. *Br J Dermatol* (1988) **118**: 203–208.

Norris JFB, Cunliffe WJ, A histological and immunocytochemical study of early acne lesions. *Br J Dermatol* (1988) **118**: 651–659.

Chapter 5

Biesalski H, Frank J, Beck S et al, Biochemical but not clinical vitamin A deficiency results from mutations in the gene for retinol binding protein. *Am J Clin Nutr* (1999) **69**: 931–936.

Chapter 6

Bonnar E, Ophth MC, Eustace FC et al, The Demodex mite population in rosacea. *J Am Acad Dermatol* (1993) **28**: 443–448.

Gmyrek R, Grossman ME, Rudin D, Scher R, SAPHO Syndrome: Report of three cases and review of the literature. *Cutis* (1999) **64**: 253–258.

Greenbaum SS, Krull EA, Watnick K, Comparison of CO_2 laser and electrosurgery in the treatment of rinophyma. *J Am Acad Dermatol* (1988) **18**: 363–368.

Landthaler M, Argonlaser bei Rosacea. *Hautarzt* (1993) **44**: 328–329.

Marks R, Rosacea: hopeless hypotheses, marvellous myths, and dermal disorganization. In: Marks R, Plewig G, eds. *Acne and Related Disorders*. London: Martin Dunitz, 1989: 293–299.

Schmidt JB, Gebhard W, Raff M et al, 13-cis-retinoic acid in rosacea. Clinical and laboratory findings. *Acta Derm Venereol (Stockh)* (1984) **64**: 15–21.

Schramm M, Blume-Peytavi U, Krüger K, Gollnick H, A rare association of multiple hereditary trichoepitheliomas with spiradenomas. *Eur J Dermatol* (1996) **6**: 259–261.

Wilkin JK, Rosacea: pathophysiology and treatment. *Arch Dermatol* (1994) **130**: 359–362.

Chapter 7

Weisshaar E, Schramm M, Gollnick H, Familial nevoid sebaceous gland hyperplasia affecting three generations of a family. *Eur J Dermatol* (1999) **9**: 621–623.

Chapter 8

Bershad S, Poulin YP, Berson DS et al, Topical retinoids in the treatment of acne vulgaris. *Cutis* (1999) **64**: 8–23.

Bojar E, Eady E, Jones C, Inhibition of erythromycin-resistant propionibacteria on the skin of acne patients by topical erythromycin with and without zinc. *Br J Dermatol* (1994) **130**: 329–336.

Buchan P. Evaluation and teratogenic risk of cutaneously administered retinoids. *Skin Pharmacol* (1993) **6**: 45–52.

Chalker D, Lesher J, Smith J, Efficacy of topical isotretinoin 0.05% gel in acne vulgaris: results of a multicentre, double-blind investigation. *J Am Acad Derm* (1987) **17**: 251–254.

Christensen OB, Anehus S, Hydrogen peroxide cream: An alternative to topical antibiotics in the treatment of impetigo contagiosa. *Acta Derm Venerol* (1994) **74**: 460–462.

Gollnick HPM, A new therapeutic agent: azelaic acid in acne treatment. *J Dermatol Treat* (1990) **1**: 23–28.

Gollnick HPM, The treatment of acne. *Drugs of Today* (1992) **28**: 353–361.

Gollnick HPM, Die C9–Dicarbonsäure Azelainsäure als neue Substanz im Spektrum der Akne-Therapie. *Dermatologische Monatsschrift* (1992) **178**: 143–152.

Gollnick HPM, Azelaic acid-pharmacology, toxicology and mechanisms of action on keratinization in vitro and in vivo. *J Dermatol Treat* (1993) **4**: 3–7.

Gollnick HPM, Melzer A, Erythromycin und eine Erythromycin-Zink-Kombination in der topischen Aknetherapie. *Z Dermatol* (1997) **183**: 8–17.

Gollnick HPM, Schramm M, Topical drug treatment in acne. *Dermatology* (1998) **196**: 119–125.

Gollnick HPM, Vogt K, Hermann J, Blume U, Hahn H, Haustein OF, Orfanos CE, Topical quinolone OPC-7251: A clinical and microbiological study in acne. *Eur J Dermatol* (1994) **4**: 210–215.

Goswami BC, Baishya B, Barua AB, Olson JA et al, Topical retinoyl β-glucuronide is an effective treatment of mild to moderate acne vulgaris in asian-indian patients. *Skin Pharmacol Appl Physiol* (1999) **15**: 167–173.

Gunning DB, Barua AB, Lloyd RA, Olson JA, Retinoyl β-glucuronide: a nontoxic retinoid for the topical treatment of acne. *J Dermatol Treat* (1994) **5**: 181–185.

Hughes B, Norris J, Cunliffe W, A double-blind evaluation of topical isotretinoin 0.05%, benzoyl peroxide gel 5% and placebo in patients with acne. *Clin Exp Derm* (1992) **17**: 165–168.

Lucky A, Topical antiandrogens. *Arch Dermatol* (1985) **121**: 55–56.

Mayer-da-Silva A, Gollnick H, Detmar M et al, Effects of azelaic acid on sebaceous gland, sebum excretion rate, and keratinization pattern in human skin. *Acta Derm Venereol* (1989) **143**: 20–30.

Messina M, Oral and topical spironolactone therapies in skin androgenization. *Panminerva Med* (1990) **32**: 49–55.

Mills O, Kligman A, Drugs that are ineffective in the treatment of acne vulgaris. *Br J Dermatol* (1983) **108**: 371–374.

Morel P, Vienne MP, Beylot C et al, Clinical efficacy and safety of a topical combination of retinaldehyde 0.1% with erythromycin 4% in acne vulgaris. *Clin Exp Dermatol* (1999) **24**: 354 357.

Papageorgiou P, Katsambas A, Chu A, Phototherapy with blue (415 nm) and red (660 nm) light in the treatment of acne vulgaris. *Br J Dermatol* (2000) **142**: 973–978.

Verschoore M, Langner A, Wolska H, Efficacy and safety of CD 271 alcoholic gels in the topical treatment of acne vulgaris. *Br J Dermatol* (1991) **124**: 368–371.

Chapter 9

Eichenfield AH, Minocycline and autoimmunity. *Curr Opin Pediatr* (1999) **11**: 447–456.

Gollnick H, Albring M, Brill K, Efficacitè de l'acètate de cyprotèron oral associa à l'èthinylestradiol dans lc traitement de l'acnè tardive de type facial. *Ann Endocrinol* (1999) **60**: 157–166.

Lucky AW et al, Effectiveness of norgestimate and ethinyl estradiol in treating moderate acne vulgaris. *J Am Acad Dermatol* (1997) **37**: 746–754.

Redmond GP et al, Norgestimate and ethinyl estradiol in the treatment of acne vulgaris: A randomized, placebo-controlled trial. *Obstetrics and Gynecology* (1997) **4**: 615–622.

Chapter 10

Ahn ST, Monafo WN, Mustoe TA, Topical siliconegel: a new treatment for hypertrophic scars. *Surgery* (1989) **106**: 781–787.

Burke KE, Naughton G, Cassai N, A histological, immunological and electron microscope study of bovine collagen implants in the human. *Ann Plast Surg* (1985) **14**(6): 515–522.

Fournier PF, Syringe fat transfer. In: Baran R, Maibach HI eds, *Cosmetic Dermatology*. London: Martin Dunitz, 1994: 421–437.

Hanke CW, Soft tissue augmentation. In: Baran R, Maibach HI eds, *Cosmetic Dermatology*. London: Martin Dunitz, 1994: 467–476.

Klein AW, Implantation technique for injectable collagen. *J Am Acad Dermatol* (1983) **9**: 224–228.

Roegnik RK, Brodland DG, Facial chemical peel. In: Baran R, Maibach HI eds, *Cosmetic Dermatology*. London: Martin Dunitz, 1994: 439–449.

Tromovitch TA, Stegman SJ, Glogau RG, Zyderm collagen: implantation technics. *J Am Acad Dermatol* (1984) **10**: 273–278.

Zouboulis CH, Gollnick H, The difficult cases: cryosurgical treatment of keloids and Hypertrophic Scars. In: Panconesi E ed, *Proceedings 1st Congress of the European Academy of Dermatology and Venerology*. Oxford: Blackwell Scientific, 1991: 417–418.

Chapter 11

Cunliffe WJ, Evolution of a strategy for the treatment of acne. *J Am Acad Dermatol* (1987) **16**: 591–599.

Eady AE, Cove JH, Holland KT, Cunliffe WJ, Superior antibacterial action and reduced incidence of bacterial resistance in minocycline compared to tetracycline-treated acne patients. *Br J Dermatol* (1990) **122**: 233–244.

Hennes R, Mack A, Schell H et al, 13-cis-retinoic acid in conglobata acne. A follow up study of 14 trial centres. *Arch Dermatol Res* (1984) **276**: 209–215.

Strauss JS, Rapini RP, Shalita AR et al, Isotretinoin therapy for acne; results of a multicentre dose response study. *J Am Acad Dermatol* (1984) **10**: 490–496.

Index